FRACTURE

ADVENTURES OF A BROKEN BODY

ANN OAKLEY

First published in Great Britain in 2007 by

The Policy Press
University of Bristol
Fourth Floor, Beacon House
Queen's Road
Bristol BS8 1QU

Tel +44 (0)117 331 4054
Fax +44 (0)117 331 4093
e-mail tpp-info@bristol.ac.uk
www.policypress.org.uk

British Library Cataloguing in Publication Data
A catalogue record for this book is available from the British Library.

Library of Congress Cataloging-in-Publication Data
A catalog record for this book has been requested.

ISBN 1 86134 937 8 paperback
ISBN 1 86134 938 5 hardback

Cover design by Qube Design Associates, Bristol
Front cover: photograph kindly supplied by Ann Oakley
Printed and bound in Great Britain by Hobbs the Printers Ltd, Southampton

Contents

Preface

This is the story of an accident that happened to my body seven years ago. It's a personal narrative which, I hope, escapes the charge of self indulgence because it's told for a reason: that is, what such stories can say about the universal human experience of living in a body.

The accident, which was a severe fracture to my right arm, became a kind of research project. When I'm not falling over and breaking limbs, I'm a social scientist. I do research. I go to the library, define a question, start a journey. My questions in the case of *Fracture* were these: Why does breaking an arm seem to fracture the psyche as well? What is the nature of the predicament of losing the full use of one's right hand because of an accident? Why does losing sensation in one's hand feel so important? Why does Western medicine treat function and ignore the patient's experience of sensation? How are hands connected to minds and self-awareness? What is the relationship between right and left hands, and how does body asymmetry work – or not? What role do 'nerves' play in the architecture of the human body? How do cultural views about women's bodies, and about ageing bodies, affect the subjective experience of fracturous events? And what can all this tell us about the general experience of being human and living in a body?

Answering these questions is what the rest of this book

is about. *Fracture* combines my personal story with those of others, and with history, anthropology, neurology, and the sociology of the body, health and illness. My accident led me to confront the intrinsic puzzle of how we can't do without the body, but would often like to. Our bodies aren't ourselves; they let us down, get us into all sorts of tangles. What happens to them, what they do to us, can permanently change our lives.

Since the accident that begins *Fracture* happened to me and I conducted the research project of this book, any errors the reader spots must be mine. Key names in my story have been changed, and so have other identifying details, for obvious reasons. At times, this has resulted in a blurring of the normal dividing line between fact and fiction. Many thanks to those - especially Robin Oakley, Jennie Popay, Tom Rivers and Penrose Robertson - who read and provided valuable comments on the manuscript. Special thanks to Tabitha Oakley-Brown for help with the children's stories about grandmothers discussed in Chapter 7, and to Tom Popay for the reference to Def Leppard in Chapter 4. I am indebted, as always, to Matthew Hough's expert copy-editing and thoughtful reflections on my writing style. My acupuncturist and my physiotherapist, who feature in Chapter 6, read my portrayal of their role in my rehabilitation; thanks also for their comments. I've done my best to ensure that no-one is damaged by anything I've said in this book; such damage is no part of my intention in writing it.

Fracture, which was a long time in the writing, was finally finished at the Château de Lavigny in Switzerland, where the Fondation Ledig-Rowohlt supports small groups of writers to get their work done in a place of unusual beauty and comfort. Many thanks to the Fondation for their support, and especially to Sophie Kandaouroff for understanding what writers need (including endless supplies of bananas). My co-writers at Lavigny – Tamim Al-Barghouti, Amrit Mehta, Ann Snodgrass and Dusan Velickovic – were a source of multiple inspiration. Our conversations about the rights of animals and humans to live in peace emphasised for me the universal, intensely perilous status of our bodies: biologically given, but subject at any moment to all sorts of cultural whims, misfortunes and outrageous attacks.

An accident at White Creek Lodge

The three of us had planned a short break before a conference in Denver, Colorado. Clare had found the hotel on the internet. It described itself as a 'Lodge', and attracted custom at this time of year with a decor of fairy lights hung over snowy trees, artificial log-burning stoves, and menus of floridly described American food – homemade wildberry muffins, pork ribs with maple BBQ sauce, French fried corn fritters, and so forth. 'Nestled in the foothills of the Rockies' said the internet blurb, 'White Creek Lodge is a quaint and charming country inn, featuring antique quilts and comfortable overstuffed furniture. There are trails for walking, and many recreational facilities, including canoeing, skiing, snowboarding and snowshoe trekking, sleigh rides and horseback riding. Antiqueing and great outlet shopping near by. White Creek Lodge is a haven of tranquillity – your stay with us will be quite unforgettable.'

The last clause of White Creek Lodge's inviting self-description proved horribly prophetic. Seven years on, I'm left with a series of jerky monochrome images. I closed the door of my hotel room, which was in an annexe in the grounds of the main building, and prepared to make my way to Kate's room, where we had organised massages for ourselves as a reward for a long snowy walk. I stepped outside onto the path which led from my room to hers. We had noticed the ice on the path earlier, and had suggested to the hotel staff that they might usefully add some grit to it. It was intensely cold; there was very little light beyond the front door of the low hotel building. The surface of the ice was dark with lumps of grimy snow. I remember putting out my right arm to stop myself falling. I remember lying on the ice. The whole of the right side of my body felt pain, except for parts of my arm and my hand which were completely numb. I felt very nauseous. Then I noticed through the sleeve of my coat that the bone in my upper arm was sticking out, pushing at the confines of the cloth.

I wanted to close my eyes and go to sleep, but instead I waited for the nausea to subside and then got up very slowly and steered myself to Kate's door, which I opened with my left hand. I announced that I had fallen over, and went through to the bedroom to lie down. Then, when Kate and the masseuse checked on my strange silence, I told them that I thought I'd broken my arm. Remarkably, my brain had come up with a definition of the event without any conscious help from me. The masseuse, whom I recall as blonde and broad-cheeked, but who may have looked entirely different, knew a bit about bodies and so took charge of the situation: she asked Kate to fetch some ice from outside the door and she managed to get my coat off. Much of this is just a blur. I lay on the floor beside the high floral bed. I could hear someone screaming. We waited a long time for the ambulance. The masseuse held my arm, which was encased in my favourite purple polo-neck jersey. At one point, she grasped the jersey with her teeth, to free her hands for other manoeuvres. I thought of it as a bag full of loose old bones, like chicken drumsticks or a medical student's toys.

This was the rural backwoods of the USA, an area staffed only by a volunteer ambulance service led by a journalist with one paramedic and another in training. As they carried the stretcher up the path, the crew were nearly all victims of the same accident as I had been. The van itself was mechanically shaky, and it didn't seem altogether obvious that we would make it to the nearest hospital, some forty miles away. The light in the ambulance was very bright; it was very cold in there. They reassured me that I'd probably sustained just a simple break: I'd be back in my bed at White Creek Lodge that night; arrangements for the conference in Denver would proceed exactly as planned; I'd just have my arm in a sling, that's all. The incident was only a minor interruption in the ordinary flow of my life.

This being the USA, the first thing that happened when we got to the hospital was that they wanted to know who was going to pay the bill. Kate's search for my insurance documents was the start of a long saga involving many phone calls, two insurance companies and the university in London that employed me. (We could all write a vindictive paper along the well-known lines of how insurance companies do their best not to help.)

Once admitted to hospital, a nurse cut my purple jersey off me. I perversely minded the loss of the jersey very much. 'Closed intra-articular fracture of the distal right humerus', say the medical notes. It was an 'impact fracture', a break caused by the circumstances in which

I'd fallen. The sanitising and obscurantist medical language does have the word 'fracture' in it, but what is 'intra-articular'? I assumed that 'closed' just meant the broken bone didn't open the skin. Interestingly, 'distal' means 'situated away from the centre of the body', a point that later seemed to me psychologically quite incorrect.

When he came into my room, the surgeon's opening gambit was, 'Ah, a university professor!'. To this I could only reply, 'But I don't look much like one at the moment, do I?'. 'Oh, I don't know,' said he. When Clare and Kate, looking after my best interests, interrogated him before the surgery, Dr Finnegan disclaimed all knowledge of evidence-based medicine, an international movement designed to base health care decisions on sound evidence of effectiveness. Most people who've never heard of this wonder what medicine was based on before the evidence movement, and they're quite right to wonder. Dr Finnegan, who fixed my arm, must have wished that it didn't belong to a sociologist with two assertive friends in tow, but he bore his interrogation well. Having established that he didn't know what evidence-based medicine was, Clare and Kate questioned him about his experiences of this type of surgery. Yes, he was an experienced man. 'I should tell you,' though, intoned Dr Finnegan most memorably from the bottom of my bed, 'that we rarely manage a good outcome in such cases'. Somehow I had gone from being an ordinary person spending a few days in a nice hotel with friends to being a potentially unsuccessful 'case'. I didn't like this turn of events at all, but I had no choice other than to proceed with my new case-like existence and see where it would take me.

The surgery lasted four hours and happened the next day, a Sunday. There was a holiday-like atmosphere in the ante-room to the operating theatre – Kate and Clare were there, and someone made tea, on the premise that the one thing English people always want is tea. Because of the pseudo-sanctity of informed consent in the American health care system, I was offered a choice of anaesthetics, together with a long list of all their known side effects, which, like the adverts for cleaning substances which kill all known germs, doesn't reassure you about the unknown ones.

The pain after the surgery was of morphine-demanding proportions. I heard that voice screaming again. A nurse said I'd had the maximum amount of pain relief, which I couldn't understand, because in that case, where was it? My arm wasn't in plaster, but tightly bandaged and very swollen. Dr Finnegan told me that he'd had to use all his skill as well as seven metal plates and two screws to fix the arm together again. I couldn't, of course, use it at all. I had no sensation in my fingers, although I could move them. I was also attached to a drip, whose purpose was to correct some metabolic abnormality.

The hospital, set in the plains by the eastern slope of the Rocky Mountains, was started by a group of local women in 1892 who knew that any community needed primary health care in order to thrive. Today it's a not-for-profit corporation staffed by more than 2,000 health care professionals and support staff, specialising in family care and emergency medicine, and housing a regional trauma centre for injuries. The Rockies are famous for their ski resorts – Aspen, Jackson Hole, Deer Valley, Snowbird – all a product of 1960s hippie culture and located in scenery that President Roosevelt said 'bankrupts the English language'.[1]

After the surgery, my fracture and I are put in the second bed in a two-bedded room, next to a person called Mrs Purdy, who is on the telephone all the time, ordering things from cosmetic companies and complaining to her daughter, whom she alleges doesn't care about her. Mrs Purdy is very nice to me. She's welcoming, and she explains how everything works. She's never been out of this small town in her life and I think she finds me and my Englishness, and my friends quite riveting. Periodically, her entire very large family troop in and sit noisily at the end of her bed, eating hamburgers and staring at the TV, which hangs high up on the wall, and for which we must pay extra. The dietician and the physiotherapist work hard on Mrs Purdy, and the young doctor is angry that his prescription of daily exercise is repeatedly ignored. A nurse marches her round the floor a couple of times a day, but Mrs Purdy, who seems to have real problems, says she can't breathe and goes back to bed to make more phone calls. It isn't her fault, but every time she eats she goes to our shared toilet where she deposits the kind of mess a simple flush won't deal with. After my first few post-operative hours, I get used to taking myself and my drip to the toilet and flushing it again – no mean feat with only a left hand – and Mrs Purdy never realises what she causes me to get up to.

I'm preoccupied with the maintenance of bodily function. You get like that, when you lose it. It's surprising how quickly you can, as a right-handed person, learn to feed yourself with your left hand. I'm immensely hungry, having missed more than 24 hours of meals. The hospital meals service includes a man with a bow tie who comes round flourishing a menu card. But how can you floss your teeth or wash your hair or put your socks on with one (left) hand? One of the nurses shows me how to manage the socks: you roll them down over themselves and then it's easy. Well, easy-er.

They are quite kind in this hospital, when they're not doing painful things to you or reading out lists of the untoward effects of the drugs they want you to take. I'm called 'the English patient'. I try to live up this image, but I prefer coffee to tea. I behave quite idiosyncratically – for instance, I take myself and my equipment for energetic walks round the ward floor, not because I want to shame Mrs Purdy for her slothfulness, but because the exercise makes me feel better. If I hadn't landed up here, I'd be in the White Creek Lodge's nice indoor pool, or striding through the snow with my friends.

When I wake up the day after the surgery, there's a large, morose-looking man in a dark suit beside my bed. He's a lawyer, what they call an 'ambulance chaser'. He wants me to let him sue the hotel for breaking my arm. Dr Finnegan, a friend of his, had called him and asked him to come. The lawyer has an agreement he'd like me to sign – with my left hand (he's not fussy). I tell him I'll take it back to England and think about it there. He nods and goes away, but comes back later to report that he's driven himself out to White Creek Lodge and examined the scene of the crime. The hotel is apparently incriminating itself by having now put up signs warning people to be careful of slippery paths. Someone from White Creek Lodge with a baby and a big bunch of flowers comes to visit me. At first, I welcome the visit as kindness, then, à la ambulance-chasing, it takes on an air of incriminating guilt.

This isn't my first time in hospital, and I do what I've learnt to do before, which is to concentrate on negotiating my route as a compliant patient through the hospital system. I take their medicines, I eat their food, I smile at the physiotherapist, I thank Dr Finnegan, I don't complain about Mrs Purdy's lavatorial habits, or her loud late-night conversations with her daughter. The only thing I do wrong is to assert my independence a little too much. I decline the wheelchair which is brought to take me for another set of X-rays. My legs work fine, and it's very uncomfortable to squeeze my hugely bandaged arm into the wheelchair. This rebellion is held against me later by one of the insurance companies, which gets hold of my medical notes and argues that, if I can walk to X-ray, there can't be that much wrong with me, and they certainly don't need to fly me plus an accompanying person back to England.

Four days later, I fly home alone first class, astonished to learn that the price of a first-class ticket is 18 times that of an economy one. A chauffeur-driven car is sent to take the three of us to the airport. The driver, a grizzly bear in uniform, spins us an endless patter of tales about the history of the Rockies: mountain men trapping beavers, dollar-hungry cattle barons, the discovery of silver in a place called Leadville, how the native Indians call the Rockies, much more poetically, 'the shining mountains'. He's so taken with his tales of pioneer masculinity that he doesn't notice our preoccupation with other matters. At least we get to sit briefly in the first-class lounge. This, like the whole experience of first-class flying, is wasted on me, although I do allow myself one glass of champagne. On the plane, I have my own steward, Gary, who takes the glass of champagne away on a silver tray as we take off and then brings it back when we're in the sky. It's a revelation to find that, in first class, there aren't any silly rules about stowing bags safely away in lockers and under seats – they lie around just anywhere, and the passenger (unlike the patient) is always right. Gary cuts up my food; he used to be a nurse in a former life. My escapades visiting the toilet with an arm in a temporary plaster cast remind me of a Peter Sellers film in which he has similar troubles with a broken leg. During the eight-hour flight, there's plenty of time for such details; I have to get up and walk around every hour because of the risk of deep vein thrombosis following a general anaesthetic Some months later, back in my former life, I advise the English Department of Health on the methodological soundness of an expert report on the relationship between air travel and deep vein thrombosis. It seems clear from this that I shouldn't have been allowed to travel so soon after surgery, but I'm glad I didn't know it at the time.

'Wheelchair assistance' notes my ticket, although there's nothing wrong with my legs; I just can't carry anything. A person to carry my bags would have been much more helpful than the hour-long wait at Heathrow for the wheelchair with its sulky attendant, while conversations of the 'Does he take sugar?' variety waltz over my head. A fleeting exposure to dis-ableism is terribly convincing evidence of the humiliation and hardships that others must endure and challenge for a lifetime.

The trip from Heathrow is grey and cold, but there's no ice that I can see. I know I'll always be scared of ice in future. Something has happened to me, but I'm not sure what. I should be in Denver, in a plushly carpeted pink-lit hotel, giving a paper about the importance of evidence in making policy decisions, instead of which I'm nursing a smashed-up arm and beginning to wonder what impact my 'impact fracture' will have on me and my life.

↓

loss of sensation

2

Our bodies, ourselves[1]

I arrive home with my X-rays and a copy of my medical notes. The X-ray films reorganise my body, the living flesh of my arm, so that only the hard white lines of the surgeon's metalwork are really visible (see Figure 1). Screws jut out from a shining metallic motorway in a series of dead end streets before the motorway curves into a meccano-like structure made up of yet more screws and plates – the complex roundabout of an entirely mechanical elbow. The roundabout rests on what looks like an ordinary domestic screw – not the sort of object you'd choose to have impaled in your arm. I stare at the films, mesmerised by the penetrating white-on-black, that magic medium which enthralled its early scientists. The X-rays have re-presented my body in a deeply symbolic way. Not only has the flesh of my arm completely gone, but even the bones appear ethereal, insubstantial, in some way fundamentally flaky, perhaps just as the bones of ageing women are supposed to be. Possessing such images of the interior of one's body, and sharing them with others, is the 'supreme postmodern gesture', notes Lenore Mandelson, who emailed to friends her surgeon's photographs of her inflamed radial nerve.[2] 'Objective'

Figure 1: X-ray post surgery

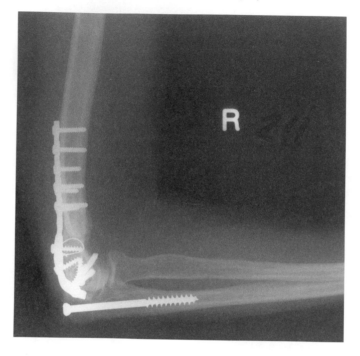

images of the body are the most definitive answer possible to questions about one's health.

The surgical notes talk about various parts of my arm as 'quite comminuted', using sentences such as 'the oseotomy was corrected' and 'the olecranon was osteotomized and turned superiorly'. 'Comminuted' I figure out, with the aid of a dictionary, means 'to reduce to minute particles; to pulverize'. But the other stuff in the notes is a foreign language, a language of insiders, like the freemason's handshake. I look at my arm when the bandages are taken off, as you would at an oddly dressed stranger on a bus. What is this? Where has it come from? From the fingers to the shoulder, my arm is studded with yellow and purple bruises arranged in neat parallel half circles. A doctor at the hospital in London I attend explains that these half-circle bruises mark the passage of the shock waves which travelled up my arm as a result of my hand hitting the ice. On the back of my arm, there's an eight-inch cut, the point of entry for Dr Finnegan's repair work. It's this that's now the prime object of medical attention. Metal staples hold together the edges of the skin, an angry red, but in places there are gaps which ooze untoward substances. The whole thing resembles a thickly encrusted modern oil painting of a bent zip fastener.

At home, my family go through my wardrobe to identify clothes that can be managed with one hand, put home-cooked meals in my freezer, change the bandages, go to the pharmacy, take me to hospital, and deal with my rages. I try to go back to work after a week, but this is plainly silly, so I get a sick note and sit at home composing left-handed emails instead. My strategy is to treat this as a temporary interruption in my life – something akin to a cold or a migraine, that will run its own little course and then move on, leaving me intact. Over the ensuing weeks, I attempt to work out a way to do most of the essential things for myself. I'm particularly pleased with the procedure I invent for having a bath, which involves sellotape and plastic bags. I can't open cans; I buy a wall can opener. I can't open wine bottles; I discover wine in boxes (not as good). These technical achievements cause general amusement, and make me feel a bit better, but through them all I am aware of a progressive alienation from my arm, which is the site and cause of all the problems. We all seem to be laughing at my arm, but my arm is part of me, so what does this mean?

One day, even my left-handed emailing fails when my laptop decides to join my hand in paralysis mode. Looking around for something suitable to destroy (not the laptop, which could be mended, unlike, I'm beginning to suspect, my arm), I throw the weighing scales downstairs. Is there a symbolism in this: destroying an instrument that measures the body most exactly, because it's exactly the body that has failed?

Over all my bandages, I wear a smart navy sling. 'Much better than anything the NHS would do,' says the doctor at the fracture clinic in London whom I see a couple of days after getting back from the USA. The sling, which I wear day and night for weeks, becomes my emblem of disability, the thing people notice first about me. Usually they just stare, but sometimes they're really helpful, like the young man in the sandwich shop on the way to work who carefully puts my change into my purse and zips it up for me. Such acts of kindness are liable to make me weep. Slowly I realise that my spirit as well as my arm is broken.

'I broke my arm,' is what I find myself saying, but, of course, I didn't. My arm was broken by the sinister ice and by what I, and others, perceive as the White Creek Lodge's inattention to safety issues. 'I broke my arm' only applies to a few people who have deliberately done it, like the American climber who in 2003, not too far away from the site of my own injury, had his right arm trapped by a moving boulder in a remote Utah canyon and cut it off, first breaking it, to save his life. This act of savagery was possible only because he learnt to think of his arm as something he could afford to leave behind. Soon after the moment of impact, when the boulder fell and wedged his arm against the wall of the canyon, Aron Ralston lost the feeling in his right hand: 'I accept this with a sense of detachment,' he notes, 'as if I'm diagnosing someone else's problem…without sensation it doesn't seem as much my hand – if it were my hand, I could feel it when I touched it'. After five days and nights trapped by his numb, now putrefying, arm, he finds a way to break the bones in it so he can walk away from it and save himself: 'I don't want it. It's not a part of me'. The psychological and mental processes in such cases must be extraordinary – the painful working through of all the options; the theoretical decision to damage one's body in order to preserve the option of going on living in it; the translation of the decision into practical, solitary, excruciating action. How to cut the arm with a not very sharp penknife. How to smash the bone so the penknife only needs to cut soft tissue. How to stop the bleeding. How to walk away leaving one's arm behind, underneath the rock, even pausing to take a photograph of the bloody stump squeezed between the golden boulders of the canyon – 'an unsentimental goodbye'.[3]

What all this requires is so obvious that people mostly don't bother to state it. Although we live in our bodies, our social and personal identities are separate from them. But mostly we assume that bodies and identities are the same. When we introduce ourselves we don't say, 'I'm Ms Smith and this is my body'.[4] We present the two as a package, since they come wrapped together: us and our fleshy, bony, physical substantiations.

The problem with bodies is that they're both material objects and the site of human experience. They're how we know the world, but they also give rise to it: 'The lived body is not just one thing in the world, but a way in which the world comes to be'.[5] What we see and hear and feel and touch and taste is all the world to us. Corporeal existence dominates everyday life – we eat, sleep, excrete, copulate, ambulate: our being in the world depends utterly on the body's *physicality*. We are our bodies because we cannot escape our embodiment. But there's a paradox inherent in this: while the body is the most abiding presence in our lives, the main feature of this presence is actually *absence*.[6] Indeed, one definition of health is 'not to feel one's body': this is more dominant than feeling well, being able to work, or being able to face problems.[7] It takes accidents, illness, ageing, childbearing or some other disruption of our normal unconsciousness of the body to make us aware of our dependence on bodily integrity.

What is the body? A 'concrete, material, animate organisation of flesh, organs, nerves, muscles, and skeletal structure', but one which only takes shape as part of a psychical and social order.[8] The body is what different cultures make it. Our Western culture assumes a particular position towards bodies: that they work in standardised ways, have a certain normal aesthetics. Bodies that don't fit create 'dis-abled' people. Certain kinds of 'dis-abilities' are more culturally and personally disruptive than others; for example, missing, incomplete and/or artificially reconstructed faces interfere with Western norms of 'face-to-face' interaction, and make the 'normal' relationship between the face and bodily identity much more problematic.[9] When something causes us to remember our bodies, we can become over-preoccupied with them, focusing on minute aspects of function and feeling, in ways that are both tragic and comic. 'Corporeal betrayal' can result in confusion, shock, anger, jealousy, despair and depression; loss of confidence in one's body may be followed by loss of confidence in self, and loss of self is a fundamental form of suffering in pain and illness.[10]

After my accident at White Creek Lodge, I have involuntary flashbacks to the moment when I felt myself falling on the black ice and feared that something fracturous was about to happen. These flashbacks all have the quality of an old black-and-white film, and the film always freezes at the point when my body lies on the ice. Then I seem to be detached from it, hovering over it like a spirit, watching to see what will happen, before the film rewinds, and the sequence replays itself again and again. This quality of seeming to be outside what happened is characteristic of such memories.[11] Traumatic memories are different from other kinds: they lack a narrative character and are often experienced directly *through* the body. The body as well as the mind remembers. Unless there's complete disassociation of mind and body (which can happen, in savage sexual attacks or continued abuse, for instance), the result is that mind and body seem more closely intermingled than they usually are.[12] This, however, brings its own terror, because it makes us – our inner selves – entirely contingent on the fate of our material bodies.

About a year after the accident, I go to France for a few days with a friend. We take the metro from the Eurostar terminal at the Gare du Nord to the Gare d'Austerlitz in order to catch a train to Blois. I have a small bag containing my money, credit cards, passport and tickets, slung across my shoulder. It's a Saturday

memory [handwritten margin note]

morning; the metro is very packed. We stand near one of the doors, crammed next to our wheelie suitcases. The connecting door between us and the next compartment opens, and an extraordinary tramp of a woman comes in, followed by two young men. The woman is heavily, theatrically, made up – white face, rouged cheeks, scarlet lipstick. She mutters to herself, brushing imaginary flies from her loose flower-patterned frock. People in the carriage watch with careful amusement, and so do we. It's an entertaining little drama. We expect the young men with her to hold out a box asking for money. She turns to face us, and I see the five o'clock shadow beneath the thick face powder: she's not a woman, but a man in drag. Then suddenly s/he and the two young men exit at the next station. When we get off at the Gare d'Austerlitz, my bag seems suddenly very light. Looking down, I can see that the zip is open; my purse has gone.

My reaction to this event is quite out of proportion to its importance. After all, my friend can pay for both of us; the insurance company will return the cash; the credit cards are easily replaced. The hotel we've booked in Blois even turns out to be conveniently next to the local police station, where a young policewoman's English, combined with my inefficient French, is enough to produce a respectable account for the records of what has happened. But I can't get the loss out of my mind. I think about it constantly for weeks. The paralysis of discovering that my purse has gone and the theatrical circumstances of the fatal metro journey produce another series of flashbacks with, this time, a rapid fire of questions: Who did it? How did they manage it? Why didn't I notice? My two credit cards were used to liberate several thousand pounds in two different places in Paris within the same few minutes. Most importantly, I'd had no sense of anything untoward while on the train. I was relaxed, looking forward to the holiday, just as I had been when I stepped out of my room at White Creek Lodge. Is the moral of this that one must never relax, because the happiest moments are those most likely to be followed by disintegration and disaster?

In her account of rape survival, Nancy Raine writes of 'neural back alleys' – pathways the brain has which bypass the control of the neocortex – the most 'advanced' part of our brain. In other words, there's an anatomical basis for the way in which situations or feelings, often of apparently different kinds, can suddenly remind and overwhelm people who've experienced traumatic events. In her case, it was hearing a radio news item about minor earthquakes while driving over the Golden Gate bridge in San Francisco: this pushed her back into her experience of a three-hour rape by a stranger who entered her apartment through an open door while she was taking out the rubbish. [13]

Post-fracture, my own life back in London becomes a mundane routine of medical visits. During these, my scar and the angle at which I am able to hold my right arm (it is able to hold itself) engage the doctors' attention. After a few weeks, they ask me if I mind being used to teach medical students. No, I don't mind; something useful must be made to come from this. The doctors hold out my right hand and invite the students to diagnose my condition. Yes, I'd noticed the fourth and fifth fingers of my right hand had started to get stuck into a curve mode, but I didn't attach any particular significance to this. Now I hear the doctors talking to the students about a 'textbook case of ulnar nerve paralysis'. The best way to visualise the posture my fingers were getting stuck into is to think of the mannered way in which the English upper classes used to drink their tea, with the last two fingers of the hand held in an exaggeratedly tight curve.[14] Because of the curve, I'm referred to the physiotherapy department, which makes me a splint to straighten the fingers. The splint must be worn day and night, or the fingers will be permanently bent. This is the first of many such splints, apparently an ordinary feature of nerve damage rehabilitation, although nobody actually says so.

It quickly becomes clear that what worries me isn't what worries the doctors. They focus on the bent fingers, the crooked arm, and the state of my scar. The most important thing for me, on the other hand (interesting pun?), is that a significant part of my right hand remains completely without sensation. When I put my hand down on a table, I can't feel the surface at all, although I can *see* that's where my hand is. My right hand is the dead twin of my left; the numb part of my hand is cold, ice-cold to the touch of the other one, like a corpse, and its presence on my body can only be detected by a touch of the living left hand. I burn the little finger of my right hand in a restaurant candle flame. I don't feel the burn, I merely notice it the next day as though it had happened to someone else, and then, with a kind of detached interest, I watch it healing slowly. At least it doesn't hurt, I joke.

I must learn to treat this part of my body as a dependent child that I have to keep watch over, since it clearly can't look after itself. The physiotherapists in the hospital clinic thus instruct me, spelling out in careful monosyllables what can't be discerned anywhere in the medical notes. These focus on the structural dislocations, the breakages of bone and skin, and the measurement of function, not on the person attached to the damaged arm, who might need a little guidance on how to relate to it. So the physiotherapists explain how I must look after my hand, counting the fingers that appear at the end of the sleeve when I put on my coat, for instance, just as you do when dressing a baby. Lepers lose their fingers and toes not because of leprosy, but because the digital numbness caused by the disease allows accidents to happen. Typically, rats consume the impaired digits. In fact, in leprosy the hands are usually the first to go.[15] This means that I now have the hand of a leper.

Much the worst thing is that I can't hold a pen. I'm totally unable to write. In Stephen King's book *On writing,* there's a postscript called 'On living' which is about King's encounter with a Dodge van in Maine in the summer of 1999. His right leg was broken in nine places, and he also had serious injuries to his hip, ribs, spine and scalp which necessitated months of painful surgery and rehabilitation. The turning point came when he resumed writing: writing is 'about getting up, getting well, and getting over'.[16] It isn't just an issue of function, but one of identity. Ever since the age of five or six, I've thought of myself as a writer. Most writers say that writing is just something you have to do, like breathing. As one writer said, 'truth flows through my arm'; it's the physical link between mind, hand and pen that's important: the co-ordination between them makes the self valid and trustworthy.[17] But this physical action of writing is also the highest form of pleasure for a writer: 'The words flow from my pen....it brings a joy like nothing else in life'.[18] I'm halfway through a book about gender, culture and the environment when my arm is broken. The book involves reading and taking notes as well as writing. Not being able to hold a pen is therefore the most complete form of self-annihilation. I'm just a broken old woman, trying to figure out a way of holding a pen in order simply to be myself.

It takes me a long time to realise that all this is about loss. I don't even start writing notes about it until two and a half years after the accident. I didn't keep a diary of events; at first, this was because I couldn't write at all, but then I entered a period of strange psychological refusal even to *think* about writing anything. I call this 'strange' because it was out of character. Autobiographical writing has a strong therapeutic function, like all creative writing. Writing is different from talking, because it creates pathways to memories, feelings and thoughts that aren't necessarily conscious. It's a way of organising experience, of incorporating threats to everyday routines and meanings, and particularly of associating traumatic events with non-traumatic ones, thereby making them more bearable. The imagination is a tool in the creation of new interpretative structures which bring the relief of closure. Narratives about traumatic events aren't simply true stories, recitations of facts; they're thoughtful impositions of coherence on experiences that otherwise essentially lack meaning. In experiments, people asked to write about traumatic events for a short period during four consecutive days also had improved immune function and fewer medical visits than those asked to write about trivial ones.[19]

It's not unusual for such writing to take a long time. Nancy Raine's book about rape survival was only begun seven years after the rape. For Susan Brison, a philosophy professor, raped and left for dead by a stranger one sunlit morning in the south of France, a ten-year gap between the experience and the telling inevitably disrupted the chronology.[20] The other alternative is to write as it happens. Admitted to a clinic in Paris for opium intoxication in December 1928, Jean Cocteau started a diary. He wanted to get opium out of his system by means of ink. 'I must leave a trace of this journey which my memory forgets while it is possible,' he wrote. 'I must not profit by suffering as if it were music, but must have my pen attached to my foot, if necessary, and help the doctors whose laziness teaches them nothing.'[21] Today, 'qualitative' accounts of illness given by patients are increasingly seen within medicine as offering unique insights.[22] Cocteau wanted his diary, 'the report', to 'find a place among the pamphlets of doctors and the literature on opium'.[23] He knew that the value of such accounts isn't simply subjectivity, but their representation of shared meanings. Theory, like everything else, starts with the self and the circumstances of experience and then moves outwards.

But autobiographical writing is often seen negatively, as a form of inexcusable self-indulgence, especially in academia, where academics repeat a prominent cultural motif in shunning corporeality as a subject of discourse: the cerebral is better.[24] Besides, studying the body is a bit like studying women, who historically have been seen as more about bodies than minds and personal identities. In a neat dialectical formula, this is why writing autobiographically is especially important for women: words, the text, construct subjectivity and therefore the authentic self in opposition to distorting cultural ideas.[25] It's also why academic feminism has itself been wary of the body, especially the sexual body, wanting to avoid the oppressive patriarchal mistake of identifying women too narrowly with their bodies.[26]

We think about losing people, jobs, houses, countries and limbs as very different kinds of loss. But the human experience of loss is very much the same, whatever is lost. Numbness, anger, anxiety, and depression are different, overlapping moments in response. I first wrote about this twenty six years ago in a book called *Women confined*[27] which describes the social and emotional losses ordinary mothers experience in childbirth. *Women confined* refers to a book by Peter Marris called *Loss and change* which inventively puts together different experiences of loss – bereavement among East Enders in London, slum clearance in Nigeria, North American experiments in social reform – and discusses the parallels in people's reactions: '...loss disrupts our ability to find meaning in experience ...grief represents the struggle to retrieve this sense of meaning...'[28] In the same way, Gay Becker, more recently, has used different 'narratives of disruption' – infertility, old age, the paralysis of stroke, chronic illness – to show how these 'moral' accounts can heal biographical discontinuities.[29]

Apart from Marris's work, in *Women confined* I also referred to work on responses to amputation, and quoted a psychiatric article on the aftermath of hand disability. It's one of those moments when you suspect there's a Great Plan Behind It All. I'm amazed and horrified that I could have written so presciently then of what was happening to me now. I looked up the article for a second time while writing this book. The psychiatric complications of hand injuries tend to be more severe than for other injuries, because it's through our hands

24

that we make contact with the world and other people. Hundreds of daily activities are absolutely dependent on the hand. Paralysis of the hand generates 'Images of death, as the withering of a plant or the drying up of the body... The claw hand [produced as a result of the kind of nerve injury I had] is a symbol of aggression looked on with fear, as if something evil'.[30]

Most of us have an image of ourselves as intact bodies – not necessarily complete ones, because not many people get to middle age without various bits missing, or in a state of some disarrangement: teeth, appendix, tonsils, bits of skin, the inside bits of women; for men, the prostate gland, perhaps, which many of them never knew they had. My own intact body is missing a number of teeth, a bit of my tongue, one fallopian tube, a chunk of my cervix and now quite a lot of whatever made up the architecture of my elbow. What bits of your body have you still got? What have you managed to do without? It's amazing what we *can* do without, but that doesn't mean we like it. According to the sociologist Anthony Giddens, the project of the self in modern society has largely become the project of the body.[31] Bodily integrity is a *moral* as well as a physical quality and all this circles round the epicentre of youth-ism: youthfulness has become the principal criterion for making aesthetic judgments about the body.

A body like mine labelled with its bus pass: what right has it got to mind the loss of various bits and pieces? It isn't the body that minds, of course; it's me. The body I live in merely houses the stigmata of loss – the scars, the spaces, the dead ends, the debris of dead tissue. My right arm is crooked, painful, weak. I don't mind my crooked arm very much, but I do mind the loss of my right hand.

25

Yes, some of it works, but it isn't the same right hand as I had before. It doesn't respond to heat and cold, vibration and silence, and texture and substance the way it did once, and it probably never will. Finally, I realise the hard truth that I will probably never have any life without this damaged hand.

Of course, this isn't a big deal compared with the truly awful things that happen to some people. Maybe I'm just depressed, and that's why I feel so pessimistic. Perhaps it's post-traumatic stress disorder: disassociation, flashbacks, hypervigilance, exaggerated startle response, sleep disorder, inability to concentrate, loss of interest in significant activities, a sense of a foreshortened future[32] – I have most of the symptoms. But who needs a surfeit of medical labels? I'm coping, though I said I wouldn't. I'm back at work. I work about seventy hours a week. I take my grandchildren out for tea. I change the baby's nappy, though the first time I do this I have to enlist the services of a friend, because only an extremely docile baby can be changed with one hand. The one thing I really enduringly *can't* do is the wretched clips on the car seat and pushchair harnesses which call for advanced manual dexterity.

I keep a list of all my medical appointments for the ambulance-chaser – that unwelcome visitor to my US hospital bedside whose laconic persistence is to dog almost five years of my life. I am a moonlighter, I have a second career as a medical patient, and I learn anew the rules and rites of that unequal career. The doctors make approving noises when they clip the X-rays to their light box: yes, Dr Finnegan's engineering achievements *are* remarkable. The doctors, lost in their professional admiration, seem to forget that the image on the screen is actually *my arm*. A repetitive repertoire of interactions develops around my arrival at the fracture clinic reception desk, where the clerk can never find my X-rays because *I* have them. I cart them back and forth to the hospital with me in a frayed brown envelope. 'Patient has own X-rays', she finally marks my record card, grinning at this resolution of her bureaucratic dilemma. I tell her (since she seems interested in evidence) that patients are generally better keepers of their own medical records than anyone else.[33]

Once the scar has healed, the doctors are only interested in how much I can move my arm and how straight I can get it. The metal creaks: if I put my left hand on my right elbow, I can feel Dr Finnegan's much-admired plates and screws. The doctors tell me that new bone just grows round the metal. It's hard to believe. People make jokes about metal detectors at airports. I'm not fussed, I don't think I'll ever be flying again. In hours of physiotherapy, my arm is stretched, measured, pummelled, discussed. I, as its owner, am advised how to treat it, how far to push the exercises, when to let it carry what kind of weights, how soon to let it loose in the swimming bath. Swimming with my damaged arm is very strange. When I look at it under the water, it's crooked compared with the other one, but what disturbs me much more is that my right hand seems to be a turtle, a claw-shaped aquatic animal that has nothing to do with me – it just happens to be swimming ahead of me in the water.

All this rehabilitation work feels to me like a chore – housework of the body, like all housework inadequately timetabled in the quotidian scheme of things. But, since it's in my nature to resist just being a patient, my expeditions to medical appointments become stolen times when I start to re-invent myself as a free-falling human being. It's a secret mission: I'm saving myself from what my body has done to me. Most of my appointments take place in an area of a couple of square miles: Bloomsbury, south of Oxford Street, north of Regent's Park. These visits become a voyage of discovery through a city I've never had reason to notice in such detail before. I find bits of London I don't know about. I discover coffee houses for the first time. Sometimes I add a sandwich bar to my list, and sit people-watching on a high stool, munching beetroot crisps or fancy bread. It's like committing adultery: this activity isn't a legitimate part of my everyday life; it isn't what I'm supposed to be doing. Nobody knows it's me doing it, and nobody who knows me knows what I'm doing, but, because of the way I manage to construct it, I *am* doing something *for myself.*

In her book *Writing a woman's life,*[34] the American professor of English literature, Carolyn Heilbrun, discussed how her choice of the pseudonym 'Amanda Cross' for writing detective fiction appeared, when she first made it, to be a simple pragmatic decision related to her need to conceal her identity as a detective story writer from a possibly judgmental academia. However, the decision to use a pseudonym was really because Heilbrun needed to create a personal space for herself. She only appreciated this meaning looking back. Perhaps it's especially hard for women, the arch role-players, to notice when the art of surviving drives them past the land of coping to another more selfish place.

My slings and splints and bandages are all insignia of disability. The first splint is replaced by others, which must be worn for years after the sling is no longer needed.

One particularly gruesome one has metal clips which have to be progressively tightened. The most complicated is something called a 'volar double digit extension splint with palmar bar' (see Figure 2); this is an inflexible moulded strap that encloses the entire palm and back of my hand, with a rigid offshoot to wrap up my fourth and fifth fingers. People are really impressed when I offer this package in a handshake. (Sometimes I put this splint on when I no longer need to, but am going to meet someone I imagine I won't particularly like.)

Figure 2: One of many hand splints

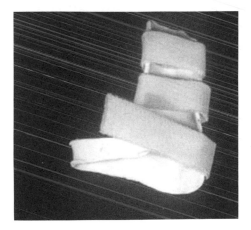

Volar double digit extension splint with palmar bar

When the slings and splints, outward signs of abnormality, finally disappear, I'm assumed to have become normal again. My hand works, sort of. No casual observer will notice a problem. It's impossible to see that

I don't feel I have a right hand. It just hangs there at the end of my arm. I hate it. I want someone to take it away and give me my old right hand back. There's even a technical medical name for this: 'misoplegia', which means violent hatred of a paralysed or malfunctioning limb. People sometimes abuse it verbally and physically. You can't include in your self-love a limb you can't feel: the dead appendage is frightening, better to objectify it altogether. 'Misoplegia' is what Chris Hallam, the world's first hand transplant patient, suffered from when he demanded that the surgeons amputate the hand of a dead motorcyclist they'd gone to great pains to give him three years before. It wasn't his hand – it was wider and longer, differently coloured, with dry, unfamiliar skin. It was a dead man's hand, and he knew it. 'I've become mentally detached from it', he said.[35]

3

Nervous disorder

Oliver Sacks fell over on a Norwegian mountain after an encounter with a bull. His main injury was to the muscles and nerves in one of his legs. A surgeon in a local hospital operated on his leg, saying, 'We'll just reconnect you'. According to the surgeon, the leg's function had been perfectly restored, and Sacks' notes were marked with the term 'uneventful recovery'. However, when the plaster cast was taken off, Sacks couldn't feel his leg. 'There was absolutely no sensation whatever,' he noted. 'It was clear that I had a leg which looked anatomically perfect, and which had been expertly repaired, and healed without complication, but it looked and felt uncannily alien – a lifeless replica attached to my body.'[1]

Most people experience this sort of alienation from time to time. You lie on an arm while asleep and wake to find it grotesquely numb, but, when you move it around, sensation returns. For Sacks, this didn't happen. He could *see* the flesh of his leg, but he couldn't *feel* it. His leg had disappeared subjectively. 'I had lost something – that was clear. I seemed to have lost my leg – which was absurd, for there it was....safe and sound...a "fact".'[2]

When Sacks complained to his doctors that he

31

couldn't feel his leg, one didn't believe him and the other said it wasn't his business. A doctor himself, Sacks explains the fate of his leg in two ways. First, the femoral nerve, which was damaged in his encounter with the Norwegian bull, had become physically less efficient at conducting electrical impulses. This could be, and was, eventually picked up by the doctors – nerve conduction tests carried out after four years showed marked impairment of function in his left leg. But no medical tests or examinations could reveal the second problem. The nerve damage had resulted in a basic disturbance of Sacks' entire sensory system, such that his brain no longer 'knew' what his leg was doing.

Sacks' description of his leg as an alien object attached to his body exactly matched the perception of my hand that developed in the months following the accident. It's shocking to experience part of one's body as lifeless flesh when one 'knows' it isn't. The limb moves when you tell it to, although some of the more detailed instructions no longer seem to be getting through. However, although you can see the limb moving, you can't sense where it is: it could be anywhere, for all you know.

The femoral nerve, which features in Sacks' story of nervous disorder, and the ulnar nerve, which stars in my own, are both 'peripheral' nerves. They connect sensation in the limbs to the central nervous system in the brain. What we're talking about here is therefore most fundamentally the mind-body problem: the relationship that exists between the body and consciousness, between the experience of living in a body and being a person with knowledge and understanding, and a distinct individual and social identity. It's a problem that has long troubled philosophers and scientists in Western culture. The mind – consciousness – is strictly immaterial: it has no direct biological representation. Yet mind and body are evidently also aspects of the same living organism: the mind is affected by the body, and the body by the mind. Rather perversely, our cultural habit of treating the mind-body problem as a dualism of opposites can pass unchallenged so long as both mind and body work smoothly. It's only when one or the other develops problems – or when some disruption of their connection ruffles their normal role-relationship – that the dualistic model begins to fall apart. Sometimes, not even the experts can work out where a particular problem actually *is* – in the mind or the body – and this also points to the flawed epistemology of dualism: we are both our minds and our bodies; they are simply classes of experience standing 'in a ceaseless interchange'.[3]

No-one in the Colorado hospital where they fixed the fractured bones in my right arm explained the accompanying nerve damage. The doctors in the London fracture clinic were only interested in what the reconstituted arm looked like externally, and in how it functioned; their interest in my experience was limited to questions about pain. When I said I couldn't feel part of my hand, they nodded and changed the subject. Out of desperation, I looked up 'ulnar nerve' on the internet. The internet has revolutionised people's access to health information; contrary to medical scepticism, using it generally improves patients' knowledge and health.[4] Within a few seconds, I was delivered a neat map of the area of the hand affected by the ulnar nerve's function or dysfunction, but when I mentioned the term 'ulnar nerve' to one of the doctors, he looked completely horrified and asked, 'How do you know about that?'.

The ulnar nerve is one of three main nerves in the hand. It directly controls sensation in the hand from above the wrist to a line running down the middle of the fourth finger and including the fifth finger and the palm and the back of the hand between these fingers and the wrist. The most frequent site of injury to this nerve is the wrist, and the most usual cause is putting one's hand through a window pane; elbow fractures are also common.[5] In ulnar nerve paralysis, there's usually a mixture of numbness and pain or tingling sensation, and an undue sensitivity to cold. Most importantly, the area affected goes far beyond that served directly by the nerve. Because the ulnar nerve is the nerve of fine movements, damage to it also results in general weakness, clumsiness and loss of co-ordination throughout the hand. This doesn't happen immediately, but develops over the first few days and weeks. The hand becomes progressively dysfunctional and this dysfunction extends to the muscles controlling all the fingers.

When, on my insistence, I'm referred on from the fracture clinic to a specialist orthopaedic hospital, the physiotherapist there points out this strange effect to me: where once there was muscle between my thumb and first finger, there's now just a fold of empty skin. This muscle paralysis is responsible for the 'claw-like' deformity that follows ulnar nerve injuries, and the need for a variety of splints. It's why I can't grip anything and can't put coins in slots, keys in doors, pens to paper. This effect is getting worse, not better. I can stand for ages on my front doorstep trying to get the key in the lock (obstinately refusing to use my left hand), and the same thing happens at the underground station when I attempt to buy a ticket from a machine, although in this case the queues behind me are audibly impatient. The skin on that part of my hand has also become horribly dry and flaky, increasing my sense of it as an alien object.

In my American hospital notes, which I eventually read, I note that the occupational therapist wrote two days after the surgery: 'Addendum: pt.poss.ulnar nerve damage? Sensational [sic] deficit 4th and 5th digits.' This language of 'deficit' is interesting. It's neurology's favourite word, says Sacks in his famous *The man who mistook his wife for a hat*. 'Deficit' means impaired neurological function – loss of speech, language, memory, vision, dexterity, identity. All these have labels, which read like a list of flowery women's names: Aphonia, Aphemia, Aphasia, Alexia, Apraxia, Agnosia, Amnesia, Ataxia – the 'A', a Greek prefix, means 'not' or 'without'.[6] Yet, to call what I have a 'deficit' is like referring to abdominal surgery for childbirth as Caesarean 'section'. The plain truth is that surgery is surgery and a paralysed nerve is a serious injury. What also becomes clear to me over time is that the doctors don't really know *why* I have this 'deficit', and that may be one reason why they don't talk about it. Dr Finnegan, who fixed my fracture, told me that the nerve hadn't been severed, just, presumably, badly bruised. But if it's only bruised, why doesn't it recover? He moved it from the back to the front of my elbow because he needed the place that usually houses it for his fancy metalwork. This doesn't explain the 'deficit' either, although I do note in the course of my research that the disadvantages of ulnar nerve transposition, a manoeuvre used to treat other conditions, aren't really known.[7]

On 25 April 1903, an English doctor, Henry Head, arranged to have the radial nerve in his forearm cut and reunited with silk sutures, in the interest of finding out more about what happens to the mind-body connection when sensory pathways between peripheral nerves and the brain are disrupted. Head, a London Hospital physician, the son of an insurance broker and the husband of a Sussex girls' school headmistress, was 41 at the time of the operation and in perfect health. His main collaborator in this voyage of neural discovery was the anthropologist and doctor, W.H.R. Rivers. The background to the Head-Rivers project was the inadequate model espoused at the time for explaining peripheral nerve 'deficits': that human beings have specific sense organs, and sensation is transmitted to the cerebral cortex from end organs by specialised nerve fibres enclosed in a single spinal tract. Head and Rivers suspected that the process was a good deal more complicated than that. Their classic two-volume work, *Studies in neurology* (1920),[8] draws on clinical studies of patients treated in London hospitals to expound their more complex explanation.

The main material contributing to Head and Rivers' new model came from the observations they both made following the intentional severance of Head's radial nerve. These observations were carried out in a set of rooms inhabited by Rivers in St John's College, Cambridge. A photograph shows Head and Rivers sitting in very serious poses framed with rows of dark books at a table laid with a prudish fringed Victorian cloth, piles of instruments and notebooks, and a jug of water.[9] The rooms were quiet, which was essential to the kind of tests they were conducting – even the knock of a servant at the door could be disruptive. Head would come to Cambridge at weekends; he and Rivers would work on the tests in the mornings, then Head would walk or ride or bathe in the river in the afternoon, and the tests would resume at 5 pm, after which there were 'many sociable evenings'.[10]

Immediately after the surgery, Head lost all 'cutaneous sensibility' over a large area of his forearm and the back of his hand: neither cotton wool, nor pin pricks, nor heat and cold were subjectively perceived by him. Other changes accompanying this disturbed sensation affected the skin, the muscle and the circulation of the blood in the parts of the arm and hand controlled by the cut nerve. At two weeks post-surgery, the skin of Head's hand became inelastic, dry and a deeper red. It didn't sweat in the hot weather of July 1903. Head and Rivers noted that such skin also goes blue 'at temperatures that produce no such effect upon the normal skin'.[11] After seven weeks, 'prick' sensation began to return and, after 200 days, the whole area was prick-sensitive, but the insensitivity to light touch, and to heat and cold, took much longer to recover. The last observations were made four years and eight months after the surgery, at which point sensation in Head's arm and hand was still abnormal.

The fate of Henry Head's deliberately injured hand enabled the two men to develop a typology of sensation which divided it into 'protopathic' and 'epicritic'. In protopathic sensation, there's response to gross stimuli and a much higher threshold for the perception of any stimulus, and such sensation is apt to be unpleasantly intense and hard to locate accurately: 'When the normal hand is pricked with a pin, a sensation of sharpness is produced almost as soon as the point touches the skin. Over protopathic parts the point must be applied more firmly before pain is produced, and this sensation not only arises more slowly, but lasts after the stimulus is removed'.[12] With epicritic sensation, feeling is discrete, localised, discriminating and informative. When a peripheral nerve is damaged, so Head and Rivers decreed, protopathic sensation would recover first, to be followed by epicritic.

Head and Rivers' theory about sensation had an evolutionary edge to it. They believed that the stages of neural recovery they had observed marked an evolutionary journey from animal to human status: protopathic sensation was the original, most primitive form; epicritic, the more refined and civilised. This theory was in tune with the times. Eugenics, an international movement which proposed genetically shaped differences in social desirability, was very popular in Britain during the early years of the twentieth century.[13] Its main scientific pioneer was Francis Galton, a cousin of Charles Darwin.

In order to prove the evolutionary scheme more convincingly, Head and Rivers embarked on a second more extraordinary set of observations. These involved Head's penis. The reason for choosing the penis was that a search of the existing medical literature suggested that the skin on the glans most exhibited protopathic characteristics. Accordingly, the two men tested Head's penis with cotton wool, fine hairs, needles and glasses of water. They found that the glans was insensitive to cotton wool and hairs, but the needles hurt. Altogether, this part of Head's body responded just like the skin on the back of his hand affected by the cut radial nerve. Of the water experiments, Head and Rivers wrote: 'The foreskin was drawn back, and the penis allowed to hang downwards. A number of drinking glasses were prepared containing water at different temperatures. Head stood with his eyes closed and Rivers gradually approached one of the glasses until the surface of the water covered the glans but did not touch the foreskin. Contact with the fluid was not appreciated.... From 0c to 21c, a sensation of cold was always produced which seemed "colder" than over the skin of the penis. Between 21c and 26c the answers were not uniform; sometimes the water was said to be cool, sometimes Head did not recognise that he had been stimulated.

'But if the glass was carefully raised, so that the water reached the neighbourhood of the corona without stimulating the frenulum or the foreskin, the same temperature was called pleasant heat.'[14]

It's a totally bizarre image: these two men fiddling around with glasses of water and Head's genitalia in the refined surroundings of Rivers' college rooms in Cambridge. One wonders what would have happened had a servant *really* knocked at the door. And what did these experiences mean to them? What did they feel, not physically, but emotionally?

As Head and Rivers noted, peripheral nerve injuries affect the skin, which becomes dry and scaly. The blood vessels develop 'vasoconstrictor paralysis', which explains why the skin round the affected part becomes unduly sensitive to the cold.[15] Muscle wastage is inevitable with all but the most minor injuries, becoming obvious four to six weeks after the injury.[16] Full recovery of sensation, and even of function, is said to be rare[17]; and there's usually some 'residual deficit'[18] as there was in Henry

Head's case. Head and his colleagues also examined the fate of a group of London Hospital patients with ulnar nerve injury: three out of five whose nerve was injured but not severed were better at 13, 90 and 181 days respectively, although the 13-day one had only been kicked. The other two had not recovered 257 and 793 days post-injury.[19] More recent studies show that motor function is more likely to recover than sensory function, but damage to the ulnar nerve has a worse prognosis than damage to other nerves in the hand.[20]

The Head-Rivers model of 'man's' sensory system wasn't taken very seriously at the time. In the 1950s, it began to get more attention as a description of the complex relationship existing between bodies and the subjective perceptions of their owners.[21] There's still a lot that modern neurology doesn't understand about nerve injury. Most importantly, predicting who will recover fully from nerve injury is still largely a matter of guesswork. Attitude[22] and age[23] are both said to be important, with young, positive people being more likely to get better and to do so quickly.

Like many scientific and technical advances, modern understandings of peripheral nerve injury are also an accidental byproduct of war. Since soldiers commonly get shot in their arms and legs, they provide a ready laboratory of material for scientists keen to explore the consequences of nerve damage for the links between bodies, nerves and minds without resorting to Head's gratuitous method of self-surgery. The classic work is by another pair of doctors, the Russians Leont'ev and Zaporozhets. In their *Rehabilitation of hand function*, published in Russian in 1945, they described 200 soldiers with injured and surgically repaired hands. Leont'ev and

Zaporozhets were interested in examining the notion that nerve injuries, such as those caused by gunshot wounds, simply disrupt the mechanism responsible for movement. They suspected, and then showed by looking at the cases described in their book, that this mechanistic model doesn't match the experimental facts. The method they used to establish this was quite revolutionary: they talked to some of the many soldiers admitted to a specialist hospital treating nerve injury and asked them what they felt.

On the basis of such 'qualitative' accounts, Leont'ev and Zaporozhets argued that, when a limb is injured, what happens is a process of 'limb reorganization'. Movement is restricted and weakened, but there's also, more fundamentally, a deformation of the peripheral 'proprioceptive field' of the limb. The kinds of sensations which reach the brain from an injured limb directly produce disordered and deficient subjective perceptions. The soldier's damaged hands or legs give rise to damaged body maps and images. The injured hand, for example, becomes 'blind' and 'strange'.[24] This is despite the fact that the normal sensomotor connections usually return quickly, so that people are able to move their hands. But what they *can't* do is recognise an object by means of the hand. 'On a tactile basis, the form of the object does not occur to them.'[25] Leont'ev and Zaporozhets call this 'tactile agnosia' – lack of awareness of the shape of an object. The hand gets lost in the object: 'tactile vision' is impaired; the hands can no longer 'see'. Interestingly, the hands of blind soldiers, which can't *actually* be seen by their owners, take even longer to recover.

Modern neurology tells us that the body is mapped onto the surface of the brain, not literally, but in the form of nervous connections. However, this is no democratic system, and some parts of the body have much more cortical space than others. The heart, liver and kidneys are entirely absent from the cortical map – we have no felt image of them. This is one reason why the pain of a heart attack isn't subjectively felt in the heart, but in the chest, the shoulder and the arm. The other reason why pains may be felt in funny places is the way that human bodies grow. For example, an injury in the spleen causes pain in the top of the left shoulder, because in the fetus the same nerve segments give rise to the neck, the upper arm and the spleen.[26] The skin is the greatest and most ancient sense organ of the body since it and the entire nervous system arise from the same ectodermal layer.[27] But by far the largest area of the brain's body map is devoted to the hands and the face; a quarter of the brain's map is devoted to the hands.[28] To be more precise, which is what modern neurology tries to be, the hands are projected in area 3B of the somatosensory cortex, and separate fingers are represented by well-defined bands within this.[29] The exact mapping of the body onto the brain is how we're able to feel that our bodies belong to us. It's a kind of sixth sense, but its importance in what Oliver Sacks calls the 'neurology of identity'[30] means that it's been given a technical name: 'proprioception'.

All this means that the drama of recovery after peripheral nerve injuries is unfolded not only at the periphery – in the affected muscle, nerve or joint – but also at the centre, in the brain, mind, personality and identity of the patient. This is why the stress of traumatic hand injuries is considered equivalent to the trauma and misery suffered by survivors of disasters, such as the sinking of the cruise ship *Estonia*.[31]

Sacks calls it 'body ego'. In *The man who mistook his wife for a hat*, he describes Christina, aged 27, the 'disembodied lady', who has acute neuritis affecting the sensory roots of her spinal and cranial nerves. She feels her body is dead. When Sacks explains her condition to her, she observes that, 'This "proprioception" is like the eyes of the body, the way the body sees itself....it's like the body is blind. My body can't "see" itself....'[32] It's one of the most disturbing connections between the body and identity: this close affiliation between body and brain that the mind has difficulty understanding and finding the words to describe. Because there are no permanent areas in the cortex reserved for particular limbs, when one disappears through injury, the brain wipes it out: the relevant cortical area is 'denervated'.[33] This hidden response is a major factor behind the 'disappointing results'[34] following nerve injury and repair. The hand may function, but the body's vision of itself is permanently interrupted: 'the eyes of the fingers are blind'.[35] Conversely, and paradoxically, the amputation of limbs doesn't necessarily produce cortical restructuring: hence the phenomenon of 'phantom limbs', first described in 1886 by the US specialist in nervous disorder, S. W. Weir Mitchell.[36] Descartes, in the seventeenth century, didn't use the term 'phantom limb', but the phenomenon was for him useful proof of the way in which the body can trick the mind: the body's deception is what produces the moral superiority of the thinking self.

However hard we think about it, there's so much we don't understand. Why do phantom limbs so often make their presence painfully felt, while non-phantom ones with injured nerves can subjectively disappear? How do these limbic and nervous and cortical disturbances relate to our identities as bodies and selves? Some body-identity connections are obvious, and obviously mediated by culture: women may feel a loss of womanhood when their breasts or ovaries or wombs are removed; a man without a sexually functioning penis, whether or not he's taking part in experiments with glasses of water, may wonder for the first time about the links between the phallus, masculinity and power. Perhaps not all types of bodily disintegration have the same ontological significance. Losing one's appendix or a tendon in one's foot may not be a statement about one's identity. But, most insidiously, those of us who start out 'able bodied' grow into and with our bodies in such a way that we don't realise we've become our bodies until bodily integrity has gone, and with it our own.

4

Right hands

Hands, or parts of them, are offered as proxies for life in many cultures,[1] but nine out of ten people, when shown photographs of hands, are unable to recognise their own among them.[2]

The hand has twenty seven bones, thirty joints, thirty three muscles, three peripheral nerves and an extensive vascular system. It's a 'delicate and complicated multisystem organization' with an 'intricate anatomy'.[3] Sir Charles Bell, who wrote a textbook about the hand in 1832, was one of many to wax lyrical about the properties of the hand: 'The human hand is so beautifully formed, it has so fine a sensibility, that sensibility governs its motions so correctly, every effort of the will is answered so instantly, as if the hand itself were the seat of that will; its actions are so powerful, so fine, and yet so delicate, as if it possessed a quality of instinct in itself...'.[4] For Paul Tabori, who wrote *The book of the hand: A compendium of fact and legend since the dawn of history*, the human hand is 'the masterpiece which no artist has equalled, no inventor has ever duplicated. All that Man has achieved on this earth,' he goes on rhapsodically, 'has been a projection and prolongation of his hands. Even as he reaches out for the stars, he cannot do without his ten fingers, his miraculous thumb, his sensitive tactile nerves. It is the clearest, most unequivocal symbol of our humanity.'[5]

Women reach out for the stars as well. The condition of humanity is inextricably linked to the development and specialisation of the hand, and particularly to the opposition between thumb and forefinger, which gives us a unique range of movement, including the action of being able to write by holding a pen, as I am doing at this moment. The way the words are formed by intention and experience in the brain, and then transmitted to their physical materialisation on the page seems instantaneous and nothing short of 'miraculous', to use one of Tabori's rhapsodic terms. The links between language, brain asymmetry and right-handedness are said to be much of what makes us human.

Hands perform around a thousand different functions every day.[6] 'It is with the arms and hands that we feel, dress, perform skills, explore our body, and contact persons and things about us. It is with the arms and hands that we love and caress, hunt and kill, disrupt or adapt.'[7] This tremendous usefulness of the hands must be why, in English, workers are traditionally referred to as 'hands': hands are both body parts and the slaves and victims of capitalism. The craze for 'scientific management' that promised to rationalise industry in the early decades of the twentieth century focussed on workers' hands. Their movements were captured in thousands of photographs to discern the efficiency or inefficiency with which hands laboured on the factory assembly line.[8] Today, more days are lost from work annually because of hand injury than any other kind of occupational accident.[9] This constant intimate participation in the hazards of an active environment makes hands terribly vulnerable: they're more likely than any other part of the body to be injured.[10] Is it this vulnerability that's responsible for the deep-rooted instinct to hide one's hands when asleep, to keep them close to the body? In his novel about the occupants of a Stalinist Gulag camp in Moscow, *The first circle*, Alexander Solzhenitsyn describes how prisoners were forced to keep their hands outside the blanket while sleeping: 'It was a diabolical rule'.[11]

The well-behaved hand is an orchestra: when it plays, there's an extraordinary co-ordination of motor and sensory activities.[12] In the industrial system of the human body, hands are the most efficient workers: a proletariat without a mind of its own that could cause revolt, and a source of labour that brings much profit. Good hands do what they're told. On the principle that you can't have too much of a good thing, many ancient gods were given a multitude of hands. 'Manipulate', 'manage', 'manoeuvre', and 'manuscript' are just a few of the words that contain an obeisance to the hand. The English word 'handsome', originally 'easy to handle', then 'suitable', 'proper', and 'seemly', unites the hand with ideas of (masculine) beauty, although the lexical link is obscure. Words related to hands are intertwined with an enormous number of phrases and descriptions in English and other languages.

We shake hands, it's said, because enemies grasp each other's weapon hands during a truce to guard against treachery.[13] Male weaponry has been offered as an explanation for the cultural dominance of right-handedness: the 'sword-and-shield' theory, attributed to Thomas Carlyle, decrees that soldiers hold their shields with their left hands in order to protect their hearts, making their right hands, which hold weapons, the dominant ones.[14] Military symbols are pervasive: the term 'splint', which features much in limb rehabilitation, originally referred to the triangular segments surrounding the movable parts at the elbow, knee and ankle joints of the metal armour worn by soldiers.[15]

The cultural symbolism of right and left is vast. The left hand isn't the equal partner of the right: 'What resemblance more perfect than that between our two hands,' wrote the French anthropologist Robert Hertz in his famous essay on *The right hand*. 'And yet what a striking inequality there is!' 'To the right go honours, flattering designations, prerogatives: it eats, orders and *takes*,' Hertz went on. 'The left hand, on the contrary, is despised and reduced to the role of a humble auxiliary... The right hand is the symbol and model of all aristocracy, the left hand of all common people.'[16] The anthropologist Joseph Chelhod describes hand inequality in Arabic culture: 'The pitiful fate of the left hand is frequently evoked, at times with a certain lyricism. Considered as weak or incapable, it is condemned to a kind of confinement. By contrast, the right hand is strong and able; attention is lavished upon it and all privileges are accorded to it. It is the sovereign; the other is its vassal; it acts, expands, exerts itself; the other assists it passively and wastes away through inaction.'[17] Among the Nuer people of the Nile Valley, young men mark the inferiority of the left hand in a particularly violent way: they put metal rings into their left arms from the wrist up, causing sores and great pain. A ring on the right hand is used to rub against the metal and further inflame these wounds: right and left are invisibly engaged in a war with one another that the left will always lose.[18]

In the *Gospel according to St Matthew*, those on the king's right hand are blessed inheritors of a kingdom prepared for them, whereas those on his left are 'cursed into everlasting fire', and must prepare instead for the devil and his angels. Most screws have a right-hand thread which tightens clockwise, since this is easier for the right-handed, but coffin screws are traditionally left-handed. The French word for left, 'gauche', also means clumsy; 'mancino' is Italian for both left and deceitful. 'Right' in English also means 'correct'; 'rectitude' and 'dexterity' are affiliated terms; 'left', from old English 'lyft' meaning 'weak' and 'useless', is sinister. In Albania, left-handedness is said to be illegal.[19]

Another association, between maleness and the right, and femaleness and the left, is almost universal: the pattern of female weakness, (in)subordination, sorcery, deviousness, carnality, impulse and general evil versus up*right*, strong, rational male authority. The Kaguru of Tanzania believe that, in the womb, a person's right side comes from the father, the left from the mother; and the accepted position for sexual intercourse places the man on the right.[20] Among the Nuer people, the husband sleeps on the right side of the hut, the wife on the left.[21] In many parts of the world, the right hand is used for eating and for other above-the-waist activities; the left, like women, for more profane, lower ones.[22] Lefthanders may be treated differently: just accepted ('the left hand is the right'), or joked about because they're 'like a wife'.[23] The wedding ring is worn on the fourth figure of the left hand in accordance with Greek and Roman custom, which was based on the belief that a small nerve runs directly from there to the heart; left hands, associated with female inferiority, are also clearly the best place for such symbols of contractual inequality.[24]

Consistencies abound, but exceptions disprove the rule. German wedding rings are worn on the right hand; in China, the honourable side is the left.[25] Traditional Chinese thought replaces polarity with rhythmicity: the cyclic swing between Yin (right-west-earth-mother-woman) and Yang (left-east-sky-father-man) governs the social etiquette of right and left. So, in certain phases of the universe, it's perfectly alright to be left-handed.

Disabilities in the right hand can be a sign of God's punishment for one's wrongdoings.[26] They may also inspire extraordinary creative acts. The pianist Paul Wittgenstein, brother of the famous philosopher, lost his right arm in the First World War, but continued to play with his left. He commissioned new works from such composers as Hindemith, Britten, Korngold, Richard Strauss, Prokoviev and Ravel, but it's the last of these, Ravel's *Piano concerto for the left hand*, a jazzy modernist piece, that's the best known. The right-hand injury sustained by pianist Robert Schumann produced an imaginative but ultimately destructive feat of engineering: Schumann constructed a kind of pulley system suspended from the ceiling to rearrange his hand, but this caused an even worse paralysis. Thereafter, he turned to musical journalism and composing.[27] More recently, technology really worked for drummer Rick Allen of the hard rock band Def Leppard, after he lost his left arm in a car accident in 1984. With the aid of a custom-built foot pedal trigger, Allen went back to drumming, producing a highly acclaimed sound which was much the same as before his accident.[28]

Most sombrely perhaps, in view of the themes of this

book, the right hand stands for the self; the left for others.[29] When we're asked to hold up our right hand to swear an oath as part of a legal process, as I was during the course of my legal case against White Creek Lodge, the right hand represents honesty and authority because it has invested it in this essence of the self. The hand is both metaphor and symbol: a 'short-hand' version of ourselves.

As hands express our genes and identities, they've acquired many different cultural functions. No two fingerprints are the same, not even those of identical twins. Although the DNA of identical twins is virtually indistinguishable, fingerprints are an example of a phenotype – a characteristic determined both by genes and by their interaction with the environment. Fingerprints started their career as an aid to identifying criminals when the first Fingerprint Bureau was set up in Calcutta in 1897. In 1901, this colonial invention spread to England and Wales.[30] Today the US Federal Bureau of Investigation holds a database of some 53 million fingerprint records.[31]

Another use of the hand is for what most people think of as 'fortune telling'. Which of us has not been tempted to try a session in a tent or booth with a dark-eyed chiromancist who promises to tell us what we most want, or fear, to know? In chiromancy – reading the hand (from 'chir', Greek for hand and 'manteia', divination) – the right hand is about the future, the left about the past. Overall hand shape reflects a person's physical body and basic temperament; skin texture marks contact with the environment; lines on the palm are about emotional expression. The active, dominant hand shows a person's search for self-identity.[32]

Most of us are born with two hands, but most of us use the right hand more than the left. Right-arm preference is exhibited by ten week old fetuses; at twelve weeks, more than 90% suck their right thumbs in preference to their left.[33] Cro-Magnon people painted their famous caves with their right hands, and the figures in Egyptian cave wall paintings are right-handed. Such artefactual evidence depicts an incidence of left-handedness that's remarkably constant at 7%-8% in different cultures and different times.[34]

Why are most human beings right-handed? The most parsimonious explanation combines a bit of biology with a lot of culture. Laterality is rather like gender: neither the dominance of right hands nor that of men can be read directly from our genetic codes. It's what we do with our bodies that explains what difference the difference makes. Robert Hertz, who wrote *The right hand*, was a student of the sociological structuralist Emile Durkheim, and he believed that the inequalities of right and left are a particular case of a fundamental dualism pervading human thought. At least forty nine different pairs of concepts/activities/objects of critical cultural importance accompany the dualism of right and left.[35] Sacred and profane, strong and weak, male and female, right and left: 'If organic asymmetry had not existed, it would have had to be invented', said Hertz.[36]

We *are* organically asymmetrical. We may have two arms, two legs, two eyes, two ears, two lungs, two kidneys and two ovaries/testicles, but the two sides of our bodies don't match. For example, the right testicle is usually higher and larger than the left. Chris McManus, whose book *Right hand, left hand* is the source of much wisdom on this subject, first made the testicular observation by hanging suspiciously round statues in museums. The two halves of our faces are different; many people have differently sized feet; our left lungs are smaller and only have two lobes (right lungs have three); our left kidneys are higher and larger; our stomachs are to the left; more people chew on the right than the left; 60% of us have right ear dominance, and those dextrous people who can wiggle one of their ears are twice as likely to wiggle their left as their right.[37] Cases of 'mirror anatomy' have been documented since the 1830s and probably affect one in 10,000 people. You can live perfectly healthily with everything the other way round. But symmetry is fatal. In the rare instances where people are born symmetrical – they have two right or two left sides   serious heart and lung problems incompatible with life are the consequence.

Some of the most influential asymmetries are hidden. It was an obscure French country doctor called Marc Dax who first recorded the lateralisation of the brain in 1836.[38] Most of Dr Dax's stroke patients who had lost speech had damage to the left side of their brains. It is the left hemisphere of the brain in right-handers which controls the dominant hand, and this is also responsible for speech. Since Dax's discovery (which was, like many key medical advances, disbelieved at the time), much work has been done on brain asymmetry and its consequences. Damage to the right side of the brain may result in people simply ignoring the left side of their bodies, food on the left side of the plate, and so forth. McManus relates the tale of a 73-year-old woman with a stroke and left-side paralysis admitted to a hospital in Bucharest in 1956. When asked to show her left arm, she persistently showed her right, and when asked to account for the other one, she said it belonged to the patient in the next bed.[39]

The asymmetry of the human body is because our hearts, in common with those of most animals, are on the left. The left-sided location of our hearts is the basic puzzle of life. Part of the answer may be that amino-acids, the building blocks of life, are themselves lateralised. This affects fluid dynamics and makes it more efficient not to have the heart in the middle of the body. Many biological molecules occur in the laboratory in two forms, but in the human body and in those of most living organisms, only one form occurs. For sugars it's the D– (or dextral) form, and for amino-acids the L– (or laevo) form. The handedness of molecules is defined according to whether they rotate polarised light to the right or left.

Why are molecules left- and right-handed? It could be chance, or there could be some biological reason. Some feature of earth's own asymmetry could be responsible – its gravitational pull or magnetic field. The right-left conceptual frameworks of some cultures clearly link the dominance of the right to the relationship between the earth and the sun. Where the sun, the giver of warmth and life, is to the south, tracking the movement from night to day means turning to the right. So, in many Indo-European languages, the words for 'right' and 'south' are interchangeable. This may, however, be more than earthbound logic; scientists have also found an excess of L– amino-acids in meteorites from outer space.[40] Theories about the genetic origins of right-handedness link the emergence of this trait with the evolution of language and the ability of human beings to dominate the planet. Left-handedness appears sometime in the last two million years as a kind of gene mutation. Animals are not mostly right-handed, like us. Although most show right-left preferences, these are evenly distributed, except possibly in chimpanzees, who are slightly more likely to be right-handed.[41]

There's clearly a lot we don't yet understand about hands. For instance, why are left-handed women 39% more likely than right-handed ones to develop breast cancer? The excess risk is much higher for thin, premenopausal women.[42] Do left-handedness and breast cancer share a common origin? If so, what is it? The mystery of left-handedness has prompted a plethora of mythologies about the diseases or special conditions people inherit along with their left hands: immune disorders, reduced life expectancy, greater intelligence and creativity. The hand is a map of life. It was literally so for medieval doctors who read it to diagnose disease: apart from the patient's narrative, they had little else to go on. Even in the twentieth century, the state of the hand was viewed by some as an important tool for clinical medicine. Among the disorders that can apparently be seen in the hand are glandular disturbances; postpartum psychosis and 'the menopause syndrome'; disorders of the pituitary system; gonadal deficiency; osteoarthritis; alcoholic neuritis; cirrhosis of the liver; gout; sickle cell disease; syphilis; and 'mongolian idiocy'. A clever doctor can tell a person's occupation from the hand. Cellists grow calluses on the tip of the fifth finger of the left hand, and the calluses of committed gardeners appear on the palm, which feels the pressure of the trowel handle. Writers get their own particular nodules, and 'The determined housewife develops a circular or linear ridge in the palmar skin from her grip on the electric iron'.[43]

The fascination with the symbolism of the hand, with its differentiation into left and right, and the secret lateralisations of physics and chemistry, is part of my own quest to find out what's so wrong about having a damaged right hand. A functionally and sensationally disabled hand de-invests the body of its cultural power. I'm weaker because my right hand is weak. The very complexity of the hand – that exquisite system of bones, nerves, muscles and veins which is so much to be marvelled at – is also the biggest problem in the damaged hand. 'The importance of a normally functioning hand needs no emphasis, whether in earning a living, practising a hobby or allowing independence in daily activities,' begins one modern textbook on hand rehabilitation, '...Injury, disease or surgical interference...do much more than interfere with grip or touch; they attack the personality itself...Only those who have not worked with patients whose hands are seriously disabled do not realise how deep the disaster may penetrate, and how much psychological trauma, often not manifest, can be caused.'[44]

This is a question of occupation as well as of personality: 'An ulnar lesion in a heavy labourer is little [sic] disability. Of course in a concert pianist it is disastrous'.[45] The heavy labourer should probably be asked how he or she feels about it, particularly since the kinds of activities that are problematic after ulnar nerve injury include tying shoelaces, shaving, fastening buttons and using tools, although apparently some people with 'complete ulnar nerve lesions manage to play the saxophone or guitar, and fly and repair fighter aircraft'.[46]

For a right-handed writer – in English, 'right' and 'write' are homophones – the flow of thought and motion from brain to paper is through the intact, functioning arm and hand. The critical definition of handedness is as the hand used for writing (only the modern technology of keyboards gives the hands creative equality). As McManus puts it, 'The act of writing is the quintessential use of the right hand'.[47] When Thomas Carlyle's Parkinson's disease affected his right hand, it was the ultimate tragedy. 'Gloomy, mournful, musing, silent,' he described his reaction, 'looking back on the unalterable, and forward to the inevitable and inexorable…since I lost the power of penmanship, and have properly no means of working at my own trade…A great loss this of my right hand'.[48]

what about drawing?

5

The daily drama of the body

Virginia Woolf made some acute observations about the body in her essay, 'On being ill', in 1930. 'People write always of the doings of the mind,' she complained, 'the thoughts that come into it; its noble plans; how the mind has civilised the universe. They show it ignoring the body in the philosopher's turret; or kicking the body, like an old leather football, across leagues of snow and desert in the pursuit of conquest or discovery'.

Woolf would have used the word 'embodiment' had it been invented then. She had a totally modern understanding of how our experience of everyday life is indistinguishable from bodily experience. 'All day, all night the body intervenes; blunts or sharpens, colours or discolours, turns to wax in the warmth of June, hardens to tallow in the murk of February,' she wrote. 'The creature within can only gaze though the pane – smudged or rosy; it cannot separate off from the body like the sheath of a knife or the pod of a pea for a single instant; it must go through the whole unending process of changes, heat and cold, comfort and discomfort, hunger and satisfaction, health and illness, until there comes the inevitable catastrophe; the body smashes itself to smithereens, and the soul (it is said) escapes. But of all this daily drama of the body there is no record.'[1]

Yet, of course, there *are* records of sorts: scattered observations in diaries; sometimes more extensive personal accounts; visual images, such as photographs; and, since the 1980s, an accumulating, though often rather arid, sociological literature on embodiment and on people as users of health services. 'Illness narratives'[2] are the stories people tell about the human experience of illness and suffering. Because the people inside sick bodies usually don't experience *themselves* as sick, a distancing occurs: they observe the behaviour of their bodies, and construct accounts of this behaviour.

The conundrum of illness and the self produces metaphors: illness is alien invasion; haunting by a ghost; being taken over by someone else. For May Toombs, who has multiple sclerosis, '...the body presents itself as an oppositional force which curtails activities, thwarts plans and projects, and disrupts our involvement with the surrounding world...the body is experienced as essentially alien, as that which is other than me.'[3] Illness is not-me, though I am ill. 'My body is both the healthy patient and the illness – I am both disease and self...there are not even two entities here, only one: me.'[4] This is a horribly difficult condition: 'It is not I who am intoxicated,' protested Jean Cocteau of his opium addiction, 'it is my body'.[5] Calling the body alien is especially likely when there's neurological dysfunction and an accompanying loss of sensation: 'The immediately felt sense of position and movement is integral to the experience of the body as one's own'.[6] Nancy Mairs, who also has multiple sclerosis, talks of feeling 'haunted by a capricious and mean-spirited ghost, unseen except for its footprints'. The ghost knocks a glass out of your hand, squeezes the urine out of your bladder before you've given the go-ahead, and invests you with a weariness no amount of sleep can relieve.[7]

For Gerald Pillsbury, the constantly changing sensations brought by multiple sclerosis are theatre, an 'infinite game of artistic experience ... I begin to watch myself, fascinated....I watch as I try to touch the tip of the index finger on one hand to that of the other...I gaze at my arm, as if not fully my own, suspicious that this may be the time I cannot pick it up, cannot close my fingers around it, will drop the glass, or may not even feel a solid object.'[8] The disease sculpts or paints or plays music on the body. The body's entertainment is about creating reality. But is reality the temperature of the water that the thermometer says it is, or what my right hand as it is today tells me?

Disease as entertainment is an unusual reaction: a more conventional one is to feel you must make the acquaintance of this unwelcome guest in order to reach a kind of 'negotiated settlement'[9] with the illness, so that the body can retreat to its former life as a more or less silent habitus for the self. Getting used to the illness may be a matter, at first, of resistance. Jim, paralysed and in hospital, persuaded his friends to bring him beer. The beer blew the cork off his urine drainage bottle, and the nurse, measuring his input and output, was puzzled when she couldn't reconcile the cordial, coffee and soup that went in with the urine that came out.[10]

We're experts on our own bodies: we live in them, we know about their rhythms, their textures, their materiality. This is not what *is* known about *the* body, but what *I* know about *mine*. When something goes wrong, it is the individual body/person who visits the doctor, so personal knowledge is of practical importance, and it may even turn out to be more useful than the doctor's, as two sociologists found in their careers as 'migraine specialists'.[11] Such personal knowledge is especially necessary in chronic illness, which isn't something that interests doctors much. It's the acute, limited condition with a clear outcome and pattern of treatment which they're taught to prefer. So the illness of the chronically ill – which can simply be acute illness that goes on for a long time – becomes invisible, delegitimised, and the person whose body has the illness has to work hard not to be seen as a malingerer, as someone who has become nothing *but* her or his illness.[12]

So long as you can go to work, go shopping, see your friends, you can live with your illness, not necessarily happily, but at least in relative harmony.[13] But consider what it must be like for those whose body *is* their work. The bodies of classical ballet dancers, for example, are art, a livelihood, other people's entertainment. You almost can't be a ballet dancer without injuring your body, and this disrupts everything. In one study, 83% of ballet dancers had had at least one injury in the previous year.[14] Pain is a routine aspect of performance; many dancers are on constant painkillers.[15]

In one of my cupboards, there's a drawing I did of my legs when I was about twelve, a child growing up in an uninspiring part of west London. The drawing is on thick, cream paper and executed with a 4B pencil. Why did I draw my legs? I was a solitary child; I had probably exhausted all the easily portrayable still lifes to be found in my bedroom, and there, beyond my sketch pad, lurked the obvious not-quite-still life of my legs. Looking at the paper and the thick lines of pencil retrieved from the dusty cupboard, I'm taken back to those Saturday morning trips made on the bus to an art shop on the corner of Ealing Green where you could stand and gaze at the amazing array of pencils; the little pots and tubes and palettes of brilliantly coloured paint; and the fine silky horsehair brushes with ebony stems. It was easy to imagine yourself as a proper grown up artist set down among expensive canvases in some elegantly lit Chelsea studio. The drawing in the cupboard is a physical sign of a childhood aspiration; another identity; the body's history. It's all these things at the same time.

In the drawing, my legs are stuck up on a wall in front of me. The drawing begins at the top of my thighs and shows the foreshortened proportions of that perspective. My legs look fatter and shorter than they were. But if I put my legs in the same position now, and if I could find the same cream paper and 4B pencil, and had I not got a half-paralysed right hand, the drawing of my legs might look much the same as it did then. I think that my legs have changed less than any other part of me, although the skin is different – both tighter and looser, like all my skin. On the lower part of my legs, the skin was subject for many years to regular deforestations, leaving the hairs now blunter and thicker, just as the women's magazines warned. There wasn't any point in telling us this when we were teenagers, just as advising young people not to smoke for health reasons cuts no ice because it's the present they care about, not some far-off goal of middle-aged health. We don't live our lives as though health were the most important thing; we only think that when something happens which makes us realise that all the other important things depend on a mind and body in reasonable working order.

Bodies carry their own histories. Look at your own body. What can you see? Places where you collided with objects and have the faint lines of scars? Are there moles you've worried about and moles you ought to, freckles that come and go, the liver spots of ageing, white bits or black bits on your fingernails, bruises and vaccination marks? Is there hair where there shouldn't be, and not where there should? Perhaps you can see traces of burns and failed electrocutions on your skin; there may be curves and sags where once there weren't; maybe your skeleton is more visible than it should be. Your body is an *aide-memoire*, a clever surreptitious record book. It's been taking notes even if you haven't. The body knows its business; it doesn't need an owner's manual.

Each of us could write a book about the lifetime adventures of our organs. In recalling our histories, we remember not just the physical symptoms as recited to a doctor, but the aura of our life at the time and probably interactional aspects of the episode too. The sociologist Phil Strong had chronic earache for years, and was relieved when the GP remarked that this wasn't surprising as he had 'funny ear passages'.[16] In *Silvertown*,[17] a semi-documentary book about her family's life in the Docklands, Melanie McGrath tells how one day when her grandmother was 17, she was abruptly taken to a local butcher who strapped her into a chair and removed all her teeth with a monkey wrench. There was nothing wrong with them. The extraction was to make her more marriageable, since any future husband could be reassured that he wouldn't have to shell out for her teeth. It's in such ways – the perception of women's dentition as dependent on the financial goodwill of future husbands – that our culture directly shapes what happens to our bodies.

We know more about the outside of our bodies than the inside. 'The interior of the body is a context for anarchy,' writes Wendy Seymour in *Bodily alterations*. 'Our internal organs may turn against us – our cells may proliferate in mad disorder, our ducts block, our vessels rupture…Our immune system, usually a paragon of silence, may destroy parts of the body of which it is itself a part. Articular cartilages may grind down, coronary and cerebral veins occlude…Valves may refuse to close, nerves cease to conduct, or more perversely they may conduct bizarre and unpredictable messages.'[18] We have no way of knowing what our bodies are silently doing to us.

In Western societies, where the body's surface is so important a marker of the individual's moral condition, scars have a particular significance as both reminders of biography and proof of resistance. They're indicators of collision, the fracturing of the skin which holds us together, by some usually involuntary environmental impact. They prove that we were there, at a certain time and place, that something happened to us, but we survived it. We tell stories about scars, using them to display aspects of ourselves.[19] Above my left eye, there's a small scar I got one bright day 57 years ago. The sun was shining on the hard concrete ground at the back of the block of flats where we lived. I was on my bicycle; a boy on his collided with me; I fell off and hit my head on the ground. I put my fingers to my head and they came away covered in blood. I can remember the scent of the air, spring passing into summer, and I can see the texture of the concrete coming towards me, lumpy and grey. It's not unlike my memory of the ground at White Creek Lodge waiting to break my arm. Twenty years after my childhood scar, when my son fell and cut his head on a paving stone in almost exactly the same place, the doctor reassured me that scars make men more manly.

Patients and doctors often disagree about the significance and discomfort of scars.[20] The doctors I saw were certainly much more concerned about the eight-inch scar on the back of my right arm caused by the surgeon's repair of my fracture than I was. I found the lawyers' insistence on obtaining nice coloured photographs of it as a way of claiming money frankly obscene, but in a culture preoccupied with the perfect body, what can you expect? When sociologist Laurie Taylor joined a local health club, he found himself getting obsessed with the state of his muscles: 'I had become more interested in putting two inches on my biceps than in food, music or politics'.[21] The effort was exhausting; he gave up when a colleague pointed out that the health club was next to an establishment called 'The Tyre and Exhaust Centre'.

This is the iatrogenesis of the body itself – the cultural illness that's taken over from that of an overdependence on doctors. Bodies are forms and products of capitalist industry, shaped by a process that's alienating at its very core. This is the fetishism of the unblemished, youthful self. Deodorised and sexualised bodily shapes are characters in a capitalist play of commercialised symbolic meanings. Fortunes are spent on clothes and cosmetics, appearance-enhancing surgery and beauty treatments, sequestered sessions in sweaty gyms, and bottles of vitamins and potions which promise to suspend bodies forever in youthful, body-able time.

The profound iatrogenic effect of the perfect body project is a sickness of its own,[22] not only for men (and increasingly women) who spend their lives in gyms, but for women who must respond to the moral imperative of being thin and decorative throughout their lives. The bodies of Western women are prone to the medically labelled conditions of anorexia and bulimia 'nervosa' (originally diagnosed in 1860 as 'gastric nerve disorder'[23]). These sometimes fatal conditions are linked in many studies to disturbances of body image.[24] Ninety per cent of eating disorders occur in women, although, if obesity were defined as one (which it isn't), men would specialise in it. All eating disorders share an extreme concern about body weight and shape, and 'an unrealistic perception of body image'. Yet what is unrealistic can also be normal: Western cultures have now reached the point where it's normal for women to be moderately dissatisfied with their body weight. So it's also increasingly normal for girls to model themselves on Barbie and other cult anorectics. One in five five-year-old girls worry about their weight, and two in five nine-year-old girls are on a diet.[25]

Women are generally more preoccupied with their bodies than men. In her ethnographic study of a hair and beauty salon in a mid-western American city, Frida Furman notes that the women who attended 'Julie's salon' talked often about their and other people's bodies, wrapping up their tales in layers of situational detail and personal commentary.[26] Women are also more into embodiment disclosures than men. Raw intimate detail upsets women less; they're less shy about describing bodily decline. This comes from experience, not genes. You can't be a woman without understanding how bodily change affects identity; in addition, women's bodies have historically had all kinds of illness labels attached to them which have produced a sense of fragmentation. Those in charge of society's most visceral activities are also necessarily committed to an involuntary study of the boundaries between selves, bodies and the external world.[27] The big trick that culture has played on us is to let men live in a state of unconsciousness about their bodies,[28] whereas a woman's body calls for hypervigilance because it's her ticket to success in life.[29]

It's because order begins with the body that the disruptions of illness or accidents can be so shattering. The American anthropologist Robert Murphy was used to studying the exotically simple lives of people such as the Mundurucu Indians, who inhabit the forests of the Amazon River basin in Brazil. Like many others, the Mundurucu operate a seemingly contradictory system of sex and gender, whereby male power and dominance is enshrined in cultural ideology, but everyone understands this is a bit of a myth. Murphy wrote a book about the Mundurucu with his wife Yolanda, *Women of the forest*, [30] which drew lessons from the Mundurucu example for contemporary American life, a habit fashionable among American anthropologists at the time: American men and women could do with more organic solidarity, childrearing shouldn't be such an isolated business, and masculine bravado should be recognised as perpetrating and perpetuating an *illusion* of superiority.

Thirty five years after his fieldwork in Brazil, Murphy published a very different kind of book: the story of his increasing paralysis by a spinal tumour. What began as flashes of merely disconcerting symptoms took fifteen years to end in paraplegia, confinement to a wheelchair, and, at the age of 62, anticipation of imminent death. It seems odd to use the word 'benign' of such a tumour, but benign it was, in the doctors' language.

Murphy regarded *The body silent* as a 'kind of extended anthropological field trip'[31], in which he used the onslaught of his illness to explore the structure of selfhood. The tumour took a long time to diagnose, partly because the doctors' tests were all normal, and they failed to listen to Murphy's own account of his symptoms. When the surgeon eventually told him that the worst of the tumour was towards the top of his spine, Murphy noted ironically that this is exactly where the Mundurucu consider the soul to be located. In the process of his illness, Murphy could be said to have discovered his soul. He records a progressive emotional detachment from his body, a retreat into his brain, which becomes the only comfortable place in which to live. As a privileged white Anglo-Saxon male, he suddenly becomes acutely aware of the stigma of 'spoiled identity',[32] and the whole distressing panoply of the cultural treatment of disability. For example, when Murphy continues to teach from his wheelchair, the Black policemen on campus greet him for the first time as someone who's now visibly as badly off as they are.

An element of alienation from one's body is part of illness for all but the most committed hypochondriac. We have to build on this faulty ground a new sense of our embodied selves. Given the frequency of illness and the commonality of this need, there are surprisingly few accounts of illness experiences.[33] This may reflect the denial of subjectivity in the medical model: who really wants to hear the details of the patient's own story? The writer May Sarton, in one of her post-stroke diaries, wrote pragmatically, 'Everyone I know must be as sick and tired of this illness as I am'.[34] Like many others, including myself, Murphy observed that people didn't ask him what his illness *felt* like.[35] Perhaps medicine would be more effective (it would certainly be more humane) if this enquiry became central. One way of putting illness in its place – a motivation for Murphy's book, mine and many others – is to explore it in order to learn more about the human condition, and especially about this essential feature of being forced to live in bodies we didn't choose, and over whose fates we have only limited control.

6

Living corpses

Living bodies are just animated corpses. The first recorded dissection of a human body was performed in Bologna in 1315,[1] although it probably started much earlier, around 300 BC in the Nile Delta.[2] Examination of corpses was increasingly seen as an essential methodological tool for European doctors. Most of the early post-mortems were done in winter to prevent putrefaction, and on the bodies of executed criminals as a sort of final punishment. However, reverence for the dignity of human beings was too strong among the Greeks to allow dissection of dead bodies in Hippocratic medicine, and traditional medicine in China and India, and in Islamic countries, forbad human dissection for the same reason. Towards the end of the 18th century, medical men in Europe started to apply to the bodies of living patients the pathological anatomy learnt from corpses. Patients to be examined were asked to lie flat, like corpses – the standard examining position, even today. The classification of disease shifted from symptoms as experiences narrated by patients to the organic lesions found in dead bodies: the real disease was the one uncovered by the pathologist's knife, not the one the patient described. The corpse remains a methodological tool and 'regulative ideal' in modern medicine.[3]

The medical surveillance of bodies as entities divorced from human identity and experience is also part of a general cultural move to see bodies as passive objects and targets of power. Clinical examination and the inspection of criminals in prison, soldiers in their barracks and children at school, all proceed on the assumption that the 'objective' analysis of bodies, bypassing the knowledge of their owners, isn't only possible but essential to the development of healthy corporeality.[4] The 'medical model' employed in modern clinical practice has been described in the following terms: '...that diseases are universal biological or psychopathological entities, resulting from somatic lesions or dysfunction. These produce "signs" or physiological abnormalities that can be measured by clinical and laboratory procedures, as well as "symptoms" or expressions of the experience of distress, communicated as an ordered set of complaints'.[5]

When doctors take medical histories from patients, they invite them to view their own bodies as objects: What happened to your body, when? What treatment was it given? What diagnosis did the doctor give the disease?[6] By the late 18th century, the patient had effectively been withdrawn from the social world and reconstituted as 'myriad sets of mechanically juxtaposed structures'.[7] This was also a neat way of dividing up bodies so that different bits of them could be owned by different medical specialities. Developments in natural philosophy in the 17th century and later added an even more anti-humanist metaphor to this withdrawal of bodies from the social world: that of the body-as-machine. Descartes' famous pronouncements on the problem of the body and consciousness – the thoughts of a morbidly depressed and solitary young man – produced the somewhat tautologous conclusion that self-reflection is the essence of personhood. Sensations, said Descartes, aren't thoughts. Feeling one's body, noticing one's location inside it, is part of *bodily* experience; it has nothing to do with identity, whose essence lies in abstracted thought. But, if the mind is ethereal and insubstantial, and the body is solid and material, how are the two hooked onto one another? Descartes knew there was a problem here; for many years, he obsessively pursued the answer in the form of the pineal gland. This reddish-grey, pea-sized structure, located in the centre of the brain directly behind the eyes, is activated by light and is responsible for regulating many of the body's biorhythms. The pineal gland has often been called 'the third eye' and is regarded as having mystical powers, linking the physical and spiritual world. Descartes believed that it's through the pineal gland that the mind perceives and acts upon the body.[8] He thought the connection was mechanical, with the mind being able to move the pineal gland, so producing voluntary action, and the sensory organs being capable of transmitting information to the pineal gland and so to the attached brain. Body and soul, he said, meet at this point: the pineal gland is the site of the immaterial soul. There needs to *be* a point of meeting if the two are to share the same identity.

So-called Cartesian dualism has been held responsible for many sins and errors in the way we conduct ourselves and conceptualise knowledge. Its resonance with other aspects of masculine culture in Europe certainly helped to create a new science of the body. In this new science, mechanical metaphors replaced colonial ones: anatomists were no longer Columban explorers, undertaking heroic voyages into the unknown interiors of the body and leaving their names on organs as insignia of possession.[9] But there's an uncanny way in which Cartesian dualism does resonate with everyday experience. One day when I went to see my physiotherapist, I said, 'I took my hand swimming this morning'. I put it like this because that was how I thought of it: I took my hand as an object; it didn't come with me as part of me. She laughed and remarked that her patients often spoke like that, as though their limbs were disconnected from their selves. In the same way, the owners of malfunctioning limbs speak of 'the' arm or 'the' leg, rather than 'my' arm or 'my' leg. There's nothing quite as disconcerting as seeing where your hand is in space – in water, on a hard table, on a cold surface - but not *feeling* it. It's 'the' arm, rather than 'my' arm which moves.[10]

In *A leg to stand on*,[11] Oliver Sacks talks about feeling in the middle of an electrical storm: electrical impulses jumped between the fibres in his damaged leg, reminding him of Frankenstein's monster, which crackled into life through being connected to a lightning rod. The impulses come and go: one feels like the labels on electricity pylons which read 'Danger of death. Live electricity'. In the early days after the fracture, I could only make my hand feel electric by holding it above my head. Later I learnt other positions and points on the hand which, when pressed hard, would make the nerve tingle. It wouldn't normally have been classed as a pleasant feeling, but just feeling *something* was so much better than feeling nothing, and I always hoped that suddenly the impulses would build up to a point where the whole nerve would come alive again. For months I believed in this incipient moment of reincarnation: an instantaneous rebirth, the numbed nerve finally unable to resist the life-giving forces of electricity, and so provoked into normal function again. I had no language for formulating any of this, even to myself, and so experienced it as a period of chaotic, obsessive iatrogenesis. What *were* these feelings? *Were* they feelings? What did they *mean*? Lacking an appropriate language, I could communicate my concern to no-one, and none of the doctors I saw asked me to describe what my hand felt like. I began to wonder if I were mad. Inevitably, I came to think that the mark of an invalid is that her or his experience is *invalid*.

'How much pain are you in?' was the recurrent question the doctors asked. It was taken for granted that the main 'subjective' consequence of my fractured arm would be pain, and that a key part of my medical treatment for a long period would be the pharmacological management of this pain. The lawyers, arguing among themselves in their offices in Denver about the White Creek Lodge's liability, had the same preoccupation. How would I describe the pain? How many painkillers was I taking? The word 'pain' was the only way these 'experts' could recognise how I felt: it was the only legitimate 'objective' label they were able to attach to the concept of my 'subjective' experience.

Obviously there was pain at the beginning, but this quickly receded. After the first few weeks, I took no painkillers, because I disliked their mental effects and they had no impact on the unpleasant sensations of stiffness, immobility and paralysis. Pain, like whatever I was feeling, is pre-language: notable for what Elaine Scarry calls its 'unshareability'.[12] Before the mid-20th century, pain played a very minor role in medical education. By the mid-1920s, a clear distinction had emerged between 'objective' and 'subjective' pain. The first was what doctors thought patients ought to be feeling; the second, what patients complained of, and which might well have no medically discernible cause.[13] Patrick Wall's observation as a medical student that the explanations given by doctors to patients who were in pain 'were overt rubbish' led him to propose a different theory, one in which sensory and cognitive mechanisms are united: what we feel and what we believe and know are the same. This is different from what we have to do in order to cope with pain.[14] Pain forces the body into our experience: to keep ourselves together, we call the body 'it' and pain, the child of an abstraction, can be thought of as something separate from ourselves.[15]

How do you describe the numbness of nerve paralysis? It isn't like having dead flesh: 'Most people would call numbness a sensation...it is the feeling you get when the normal feeling of touch is not working properly'.[16] Gerald Pillsbury, with multiple sclerosis, tries to describe the sensation in his feet: 'I might start by saying that my feeling there has changed considerably from what I remember it being ten or fifteen years ago and go on that I experience tingling, sometimes burning, sometimes a deadening heavy sensation.'[17] 'Loss of feeling' is the phrase that comes most easily to mind, but this is a gross oversimplification, because, rather than loss, there's a buzz of diffuse sensations, so confusing that they occupy one constantly. Amputees have a similar problem: there's no language, other than that of pain, for describing what having an artificial limb fitted feels like. Different prostheses 'feel' very different, but the person in the amputated body has to develop her or his own metaphors for communicating how, for example, one artificial foot feels more 'foot-like' than another.[18]

It's with a sense of triumph that I finally locate a medical paper with 'tingling' in its title. 'Tingling' I read isn't painful; it's a slightly uncomfortable sensation that patients usually compare with electricity. Yes!, I think, here's someone who knows what he's talking about. The authoritative tone continues: tingling is a sign of nerve regeneration, technically the process of new axons growing. The more this happens, the more tingling you get, but tingling stops after eight to ten months.[19] A mythology of precise time is characteristic of the medical approach, but what is it based on? I've had six plus years of tingling, and there's no sign of it stopping. Another such mythology, present in the textbooks[20] and relayed to me by several of that doctors I saw, is that nerves regenerate at the rate of one millimetre per day. One doctor even got a tape measure out and assessed the distance on my arm this regeneration process would have to cover: in thirty weeks, he predicted cheerfully, all would be well. The thirty weeks came and went, and there was no noticeable difference. It's now over 342 weeks, so I suppose that's it. There surely can be no exact science of the body without this most authentic element: what the person who lives in the body knows.

After the first months, my hand alternated between more-or-less total numbness and a kind of dim, background 'pins and needles' feeling. There was a period when I would get odd shooting pains in my palm and fingers, sometimes after exercising the hand, sometimes not, and these, I observed, would often be followed by an incremental enhancement of my hand's capacity to notice what it was doing. But I thought of this as a *hand* problem, not a *brain* one – the phenomenon felt very localised in the apparatus of the nerve. It was Sacks' electricity, reminiscent of mechanical monsters brought to life by lightning. The main medical approach to assessing these odd sorts of sensation is through nerve conduction tests. The patient goes to a specially equipped room and is attached to electrodes. One electrode stimulates the nerve with a mild electric shock, and other electrodes record the resulting electrical activity. The distance between the electrodes, and the time it takes for the electrical impulses to travel between them, are used to calculate the efficiency of the nerve. Such tests are the mechanical model of the body *par excellence*; the patient doesn't have to speak, or even, really, be conscious at all. The tests proceed on the simple assumption that '…a stimulant current, applied through surface or needle electrodes, evokes a sensory action potential that is self-propagated by the nerve, and is recorded at some distance in either direction along the nerve'.[21] The results are judged using standardised scales, commonly the British Medical Research Council scale, originally introduced in 1954.[22] The lower points on the scale define 'unsatisfactory', and the higher ones 'satisfactory', recovery. According to one textbook, *The paralysed hand*, 'Electrical testing of motor response and nerve conduction has contributed significantly to our knowledge of nerve function and regeneration. It is…quite impressive to both patient and physician.' Patients like it because of its aura of 'superscience' and 'electronic gadgetry'; doctors approve because the test results 'are given quantitatively in milliseconds with quite an impressive array of figures.'[23]

The limitations of such tests are most powerfully illustrated in a story told by Sacks. A 28-year-old French woman was interred in the Salpêtrière hospital in Paris in the early 1900s, complaining of 'insensibility'. She said she was no longer aware of her limbs, head, or hair, had no sense of taste or smell, and couldn't feel cold: 'I have to touch myself constantly in order to know how I am'.[24] Functional tests showed normal sensitivities to touch, heat and cold, and normal smell and taste, conflicting with the patient's own account. Sensation – the physical discharge of skin receptors when a stimulus is applied – isn't the same thing as sensibility, which is the 'cortical interpretation' of the stimulus: what the owner of the stimulated body feels.[25]

I had four sets of nerve-conduction tests at three different hospitals. The early ones showed impaired sensation to light touch and a 'severe ulnar deficit' at, or around, the right elbow. The last provided evidence of some 'objective' recovery, but continuing abnormality for touch and vibration, the experience of heat as pain, and hypersensitivity to cold. The tests said nothing about sensibility – about what I felt.

Physiotherapists have relatively low status among health care workers, but they play a major role in the 'rehabilitation' of patients for whose conditions there are no obvious medical solutions. Nerve-conduction tests are inadequate ways of assessing sensation, but something nonetheless has to be done with the patient who sticks to her or his story that lack of sensation is the problem. This form of rehabilitation is called 're-education'. The textbook rationale for re-education is that 'the motivated patient who has a sensory deficit can be trained by making use of learning principles (i.e. attention, feedback, memory, and reinforcement) to maximise function in the hand…the patient can learn to correctly decode the altered messages sent to the brain'.[26] Re-education is about learning the new language spoken by the hand,[27] 'representational remodelling',[28] re-programming the 'brain computer',[29] or reorganising the brain's 'cortical map'.[30] The brain's map of the body has some flexibility: damage to one part of the body may not only wipe out that part of the brain map, but teach other parts to change. For example, some of the brain's auditory area in congenitally deaf people is reallocated for visual use. The reading finger of blind people who read Braille has an extremely large representation in the tactile parts of the brain.[31] When fingers are amputated, rather than over-used for reading, the cortical representation of the adjacent intact finger expands to fill the vacated space, like greedy relatives who grab any opportunity to have the house to themselves.[32] Significantly, of course, metaphors of reorganising or re-programming the brain bypass the person: it's the cortex, not the self, that's the object of the exercise. Rehabilitation work is work on the body, but this focus perpetuates the very problem it seeks to solve.[33]

Still, to reach the cortex, rehabilitation workers must confront the whole patient. Theresa, the occupational therapist I'm finally sent to see, is a specialist in hands. She and her colleagues operate in a crowded under-resourced space stuffed with sagging teddy bears (for child patients) and cupboards from which they magic a wonderful array of technical aids, despite lack of funds. When I was first referred to Theresa, my arm was free from its sling and holding pens again. It wasn't straight, and the elbow often hurt, but my main 'complaint' was the lack of sensation in my hand and the fact that I couldn't do very much with it.

Theresa sets to with great passion and determination to do what she can. First come several more splints to replace the tortuous contraptions provided by the fracture clinic which she says were quite wrong. Then she makes me one for the palm of my hand. I hadn't noticed until she pointed it out to me, but one consequence of damage to the ulnar nerve is that you lose the concave shape of your palm. Palms aren't flat, you need the concavity to work the fingers. So the palm splint, worn most of the time for several months, enables me to separate my fingers again. That's how I start writing this book, sitting in the British Library wearing my palmar splint, which makes my handwriting just about legible, even if it attracts some curious attention.

I am also given lots of exercises to do. At first, these involve rubber balls of various consistencies, all colour-coded, and lengths of stretchy stuff made of rubber latex, similarly coloured. I'm pleased to graduate from yellow (easy) to red (more difficult) to green (even more difficult). Some of the exercises involve plunging my hand into bowls of lentils or rice or peas, or brushing it against differently textured fabrics – swathes of velvet, silk, linen, and wool. All this is designed to restore my hand's old ability to tell what kind of thing it's touching, instead of being told by me.

There's no end to Theresa's inventiveness: she follows the precept that 'If it works for you and your patient, use it'.[34] I'm sent out to buy Chinese metal jingly balls and later golf balls, and one set of exercises requires a tin weighing in the region of 450 grams (organic baked beans = 420 grams). On one occasion, when Theresa asks me what I still can't do, I give her a list, ending with 'Oh, and I can't open a taxi door'. The handles on the doors of black taxis in London require a particular strength in the thumb and forefinger, which is only notable in its absence. 'Ah,' she says thoughtfully. The next time I go, she digs into her handbag and produces with a flourish what she calls my 'cab door exercise'. To make it – a short pole with an excrescence at the side (see Figure 3) – she's enlisted the help of her husband, who's in the building trade. I take my cab door exercise home with enormous joy and spend my evenings practising it – this pitiful preoccupation is what illness does to you. A few weeks later, a taxi driver must have been completely mystified to hear this woman climbing into the back of his taxi shouting, 'I did it!'.

Figure 3: The cab door exercise

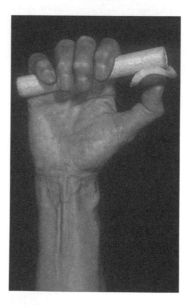

Theresa makes maps of my hand, using a modern variant of the Head-Rivers technique (see Figure 4). The maps are coloured red, green and blue, depending on what I detect different parts of my hand feel when she tests them with filaments of different thicknesses. The filaments are hairs of different diameters glued to wooden rods, another apparatus of

Figure 4: Hand map, eight months post-accident

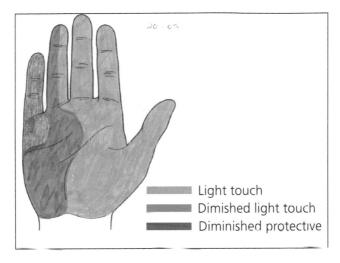

quantification devised in the 1880s by someone called von Frey.[35] He distinguished the different cutaneous senses as touch, warmth, cold and pain, and said each had its own specialised projection system into the brain.[36] During these tests, I turn my head away and close my eyes. Henry Head, in his hand and penile experiments a hundred years ago found this the best way of getting 'correct' answers.[37] The test doesn't work if the table vibrates or there's too much noise (hence at least some of Henry Head's nervousness about servants). Your senses are connected, so, in the presence of other perceptive distractions, it's difficult to tell what you/your limb is really feeling.

My hand exists in its coloured representation in Theresa's file. It still doesn't exist in my head. Theresa diagnoses the 'proprioceptive deficit' of the textbooks, which means we must do our best to persuade my brain that it still has a right hand. I feel like a geographer, recharting old territory in a new way, but geography was never my strongest subject. I'm one of those spatially blind people to whom east and west make no sense. Perhaps this accentuates my present mental inability to notice where my hand is on my body.

Enter a whole new array of material aids. On the precept that the brain needs to be reminded the hand is there, Theresa equips me with lycra gloves, made in China, with and without fingers, and with tubigrip compression bandages, to be worn the whole length of the arm for as much of the day as I can bear them. The gloves are for the night and when it's cold. They have the same function as the tubigrip bandages, but they also help to keep moisturising cream in contact with the very dry skin which covers the affected part of my hand – another symptom of nerve damage. Sometimes I laugh at myself with all this equipment, but I don't care. The first winter Theresa offers me a special plaster to wrap around my little finger when I go out. Without the plaster, the finger rapidly goes white and sticks out at an immovable angle. The paradox is the coexistence of the two feelings: intense cold *and* numbness. I try all sorts of gloves and can never find any that keep my right hand warm. Like the geography problem, this coldness has a biographical consistency: for as long as I can remember, I've had horribly cold hands and feet. My elder daughter finally finds me a solution in a sports shop: little packages of charcoal which, when shaken, give off heat to warm the hands of mountaineers. There are also little plastic sacs of gel with ingenious on/off buttons, but these require saucepans of hot water, and so are altogether more of a performance.

Most of the progress is far too slow for me to notice, despite the fact that the borders of the colours on Theresa's hand maps shift slightly over the weeks and months. This is what makes me wonder about 'alternative medicine'. I'd never had acupuncture, but it seemed intuitively possible that whatever is preventing the recovery of my ulnar nerve might be aided by an approach based on the principle that a healthy body is marked by the free flow of energy through it. I'm also attracted (on the basis of total ignorance) by the idea of needles stimulating what I think of, à la Sacks, as electrical activity.

In the UK, acupuncture is the most commonly used of all alternative medical treatments: about 7% of adults have had it, which adds up to some three million acupuncture treatments a year.[38] When I first went to an acupuncturist, I explained that I didn't really want to understand the theory; I just wanted the results. I didn't especially believe it would work, and, if acupuncture is one of those treatments where the patient's belief in therapeutic efficiency is critical, then we'd both be disappointed.

The first few sessions with Niran Samak, my chosen practitioner, do no apparent good at all. Since I'm paying £50 a time, I'm more disgruntled than I might otherwise have been. However, it's undoubtedly very restful, lying there on Niran's couch with my eyes shut, listening to the restricted cadences of taped Indian music. Niran himself sits silently, taking notes or moving so quietly in and out of the room that I'm only aware of his movements because the flow of air round the couch changes. I've never met anyone who could move so imperceptibly, and he's tall, over six feet, more with the white turban he wears to complete his healing outfit, which is designed to counter his native middle-class Englishness.

Niran puts the needles in both my feet, both my hands and sometimes my head as well. He uses light treatment to boost the needles' effects. A natty little chrome lamp is focused on the needles in my right hand, and light is channelled through jewels. This 'gem therapy' is another ancient healing system, derived from over 5,000 years' experience of the medicinal properties possessed by the earth's gemstones. Electronic gem therapy lamps, such as the one used by Niran, pulse energy at different frequencies through high quality gems, thus amplifying what are thought to be the stones' inherent vibrational healing powers. Different stones are recommended for different health problems. My hand is treated to diamond and orange carnelian light, said to produce stimulating, warm bio-energy, activity and circulation. It's the iron oxide that gives carnelian its bright colour, and most carnelian used these days is stained chalcedony from Brazil or Uruguay – though the best stuff is said to come from India.[39] I like the feeling I get in my hand from a combination of the needles and the carnelian light, but, rather than being cooling, it's a bit like putting my hand on a sunbed. After a few minutes, I get this sensation of warmth in the affected part of my hand and then the fingers start moving, agitating themselves back and forth, quite beyond my control. My brain observes what my hand is doing and thinks, 'How interesting'. After the session, I take my warm hand home on the bus, nursing it like a prize, happy at how it feels a little bit more like part of me again. I probably grin inanely at my prize all the way home, as though I've been on a very successful shopping expedition – which I have!

After several months of all these attentions, I have a conversionary moment. Walking down a street, I suddenly feel this very odd sensation in the numbed part of my hand. It's disconcerting, quite worrying in fact; but, when I look down at my hand, I can see that all I'm feeling is the quite wonderful ordinary sensation of raindrops falling on my hand. Presumably the improved functioning of the nerve has increased the sensibility of the skin, but my brain can't recognise this very ordinary sensation without some help from me.

We may experience the world through our bodies, but our bodies alone can't tell us what the experience means. When Mike May, blinded in a childhood accident at the age of three, recovered his sight through surgery forty years later, he had enormous trouble working out what he was seeing. Something orange on a baseball court was probably a ball, but it didn't look round to him. He could recognise his wife only from her hairstyle and the clothes she wore. The expressions on people's faces eluded him most of the time (his own face was nearly expressionless). Mike kept a diary recording his re-introduction to a sighted world. Six weeks after the surgical bandages were removed, he wrote: 'I have been noticing some discomfort when I use the phrase, "Nice to see you". I have always used that word quite comfortably. This phrase means much more than just nice to see you with my eyes. It means good to be with you again; nice to be in your presence; nice to hear you; etc. Now, when I say, "Nice to see you", everyone takes it literally. Suddenly the phrase is one dimensional instead of multi dimensional.'[40] Laboratory tests showed lack of activity in some of the areas of Mike's brain that process visual information.[41] Seeing for blind people can so disrupt their normal tactile understanding of the world that they feel, paradoxically, lost: a third of those who have their vision 'restored' prefer to be blind, living in dark rooms and walking with their eyes shut.[42]

Each time, the acupuncture's magic fades after a couple of days, but there is progress. I seem to be getting the muscles back in my hand. This is what the textbooks and the great nerve man at the specialist orthopaedic hospital to which I'm referred say never happens. Mr Elmwood, dapper, silver-haired and respectful, sees me when I insist to the fracture clinic doctors that I can't be cured if I still can't feel my right hand. He at first thinks there's surgery he could do, and then later dismisses this when he sees the results of the acupuncture. The last time I see him, his departing words are, 'Give my best wishes to your acupuncturist'. Theresa's so impressed she asks if she can come with me to observe an acupuncture session. She watches the involuntary busyness of my hand when Niran's put his needles in, and she talks to him about my ulnar nerve and her understanding of what's going on. He talks to her about chi and yin and yang, and I see her nodding and grow silent at this clash of paradigms. The episode reminds me of a visit I made to China twenty three years ago, with a deputation of scientists from the World Health Organization, to meetings about maternity care. In the hospitals we visited, we saw the proponents of Western and Chinese medicine standing either side of patients' beds, discussing with each other and with the patients which particular treatments from either paradigm to try.

A key precept of acupuncture is the inseparability of mind and body. The theory underlying acupuncture conceives a radically different relationship from Western medicine between the mind and the body. Most modern acupuncture is based on ancient Chinese thinking: that a critical constituent of the body is an energy force called 'chi'. Chi circulates throughout the body to nourish and protect all the tissues. Acupuncture activates and balances the chi and so prevents or treats illness. Very thin needles are placed in the acupuncture points, which are small dots on the 14 major channels – meridians – within which the chi circulates. A striking correspondence has been noted between traditional acupuncture points and physiological features, such as peripheral nerve junctions.[43]

At Theresa's suggestion, I start to play the piano for physiotherapy. I begin with simple exercises: moving the thumb and each finger up and down slowly on the keys. A colleague at work who's a musician brings me an exercise to practise: a set of chromatic broken chords, which is particularly good for the individual movement of my affected fingers. Then I go back to the old scales and broken chords of my childhood, the tatty scale and exercise books kept for forty odd years. The apposite term 'broken chords' isn't lost on me. I feel like a child again, playing those scales. I'm back in the stuffy front room in Acton with Mrs Poon, my fussy piano teacher, and her tall skinny husband with sticking out ears, who waters the garden outside the fake mullioned windows, while his wife drills me in child-adapted versions of the classics and as many broken chords as she can fit in.

I develop a routine for this, as for everything else: each night on the way to bed I sit in the darkness and play one contrary motion scale in C with both hands, then a rising octave of scales with the right hand and a similar set of broken chords, both major and minor. The darkness helps me to focus on the relationship between my brain and my hand. This is all okay as long as I think of it as physiotherapy, but if I think of it as music I get upset. What I can do now is so much less than I'd been able to do once. A 74-year-old man, disabled by a stroke, when interviewed for Gay Becker's study of *Disrupted lives* put it like this: 'My hand – this is the awful part. I try to work with it every day but it's awfully difficult. One thing has killed me, broke my heart – that I can't play the piano any more. I loved it better than anything.'[44]

I can hear my hand hitting the right or wrong note, but I have little sense of where my hand is, and the contact between my fourth and fifth fingers and the piano keys is an abstract concept. But then an interesting thing happens. One evening, I'm brave enough to put the light on and try some real music. I play some Mrs Poon Grade 4 pieces. Not very difficult ones, but ones I'd played a lot and had been fond of. One of them, an 'Andante sostenuto' from Mendelssohn's *Christmas pieces*, had a particular symbolic significance because I'd played it every morning before all my school exams. And when I play these tunes now, forty-five years later, with my damaged hand, the familiarity of the music brings some sensation back to my hand. It's as though old pathways between the brain and the body – between 'me' and 'it' – are being retrodden, causing electrical impulses to flow where before they've been blocked. Nothing of the kind happens when I play new music. I struggle with the notes, but whether I get them right or wrong makes no difference to what my hand feels.

There is, and remains, this paradox: I don't *feel* normal, although I am, apparently, cured. Classical neurology is based on the concept of function, not on that of 'subjective' perception. Restoration of *function* is what counts, and it's perfectly compatible with a continuing impairment of *sensation*, and of the brain's ability to recognise the repair that's occurred in the damaged limb. This approach fits the body-as-machine model of Western medicine, and the unimportance of what Virginia Woolf called 'the creature within'.[45] It helps to explain why there's been much more research into motor function than into sensibility, despite the fact that, without sensation, the hand is virtually useless. This is why tests of functional ability are a poor guide to what people with damaged hands can actually do.[46] Medical scientists know very little about the relative importance of these two sorts of factors they've identified as important: the peripheral (what happens in the hand) and the central (what happens in the brain).[47] Perhaps the missing link has something to do with the person.

In any case, what is 'normal'? When my left hand was assessed as a comparison in the nerve conduction tests, it was clear that all the measurements on my right hand were grossly *abnormal* for me. My feeling that I'm being left out of all this medical appraisal of my condition is confirmed when I'm sent copies of my medical notes because of the legal case against White Creek Lodge. One letter from the London fracture clinic to my GP asserts that I have 'no particular complaints'. I don't recall anyone ever asking me about the many 'complaints' I did have. Another such letter notes that I have developed a 'valgus deformity' (a bony lump on the inside of my elbow), but that, 'cosmetically', I am 'accepting'. Accepting of what? None of the doctors ever asked me how I felt. They looked at my arm and my hand, and assessed the function of both, according to their own 'objective' tests, but they never inquired what they felt like to me or what it was like to live in a body with these disabilities. Thus, it was perfectly alright to discharge me as 'cured' eleven months after the fracture when X-rays showed my bones had mended. There was nothing more the doctors could or should do.

The second point at which I'm told I'm cured is when Theresa reviews my notes and my hand, and then congratulates me on having regained an impressive degree of normality. 'It may look normal to you,' I say, 'but it doesn't *feel* remotely normal to me. In fact, a lot of the time I can't *feel* it at all.' Theresa has no way of knowing that I can't feel my hand unless I tell her. Yes, she has her coloured maps, but these only chart my brain's ability to distinguish when something is being prodded against my hand; they don't describe what I feel. The difference is that Theresa listens when I tell her; she isn't a machine. Afterwards, when we discuss it, she says that my articulateness as a middle-class patient (she doesn't put it quite like that) is what makes her listen. When Jean Cocteau was in a clinic for opium addiction, he asked one of his doctors why he spent so much time treating him. The doctor said 'that he at least had a patient who talked, that he learnt more from me, being capable of describing my symptoms, than at the hospital'.[48]

Theresa's attentiveness (for whatever reason) means that together we have overturned the teaching about ulnar nerve paralysis in the textbooks. Much more is possible through 're-education' than they say it is. Her final experiment with me is the use of mirrors to deceive my brain into thinking the 'bad' hand is in fact the 'good' one. It's a technique that was first used to reduce the pain of amputated limbs: the image of a normal limb is superimposed on the amputated one using a mirror, and pain goes down.[49] Theresa gives my bad hand a task to do which it can't, and then she sets up a mirror and asks me to try again. My eyes, looking in the mirror, tell my brain that the bad hand is the good one, and so the task can be done.

It seems such an easy trick. But who or what is deceiving whom or what here? Can the relationship between the eye and the brain be so direct, so ignorant of the knowledge that I have, as the person who owns all these body parts, that there's a deception going on? And then it seems that this transition from one side of the body to the other is something that the body can do all on its own. About three years after the fracture, I start to wake up in the mornings with *both* hands numb. The numbness in the undamaged hand is in exactly the same area as in the damaged one. The difference is that, when I wiggle my fingers, sensation returns in one hand and not in the other. My left hand appears to have developed some sort of couvade syndrome: like the partners of women in some societies who have labour pain, it's come out in sympathy. Then my left hand goes further and develops osteoarthritis – again, in just that part of the hand that is affected by the nerve problem in the right. 'Of course', says my acupuncturist, when I tell him. Everyone else just thinks I'm mad. What the left hand is doing must be completely independent of what's happened to the right. But a little more probing in the library shows that this ability of the body to symmetricise symptoms is well-known in diseases such as rheumatoid arthritis and psoriasis, even though nobody can explain *how* it happens.[50]

Theresa, the listening physiotherapist, turns what she's done for me (what we've done together) into some lessons for other people: 'Rehabilitation of an ulnar nerve lesion following elbow fracture: a single case study' is given at a conference in Ireland on 'Integrated Musculoskeletal Trauma'.[51] The presentation is a nice mixture of clinical observations and quotations from me, with plenty of PowerPoint pictures of my arms and hands doing things not very well with pieces of latex and wire, and tins of baked beans. Her summary slide includes a statement and a question. The statement says that repair of a nerve can never be perfect. The question is the one that my fracture has made me puzzle over long and hard: why do they call perceiving touch and pain sensation, when you can do both and yet have no sense of having a hand? The more fundamental question here is why the models of the body on which Western medicine depends so distort the human experience of living in a body.

7

Old bones

As a child, I used to lie in bed waiting for my mother to say goodnight to me. It was a time of day quite as agonising in its own small way as Proust's nightly longing for his mother's kiss, but, unlike Proust's anticipation, mine prompted distracting observations about gender, ageing and the body. My mother's knees creaked. That's how I knew when to expect her arrival in my bedroom. Like an aeroplane coming in to land, the noises were at first distant and then louder and then very loud, until they stopped as she cruised down the corridor to my room. This was the difference between my mother and my father coming to say goodnight: one creaked and the other didn't. So was there something about women getting older that meant their knees creaked?

Some story about women, ageing and bones is inevitably prompted by a fracture such as the one I (then a 57-year-old woman) incurred at White Creek Lodge. Old women break their bones because the skeleton, some 10%-15% of our body weight, is living tissue. Our skeletons live and die, and prosper or not, just like the rest of us. Bone loss begins in the thirties, after which the fate of our skeletons is all downhill. This is true for men as well as women, but women's skeletons also have to deal with the withdrawal of bone-protecting hormones at the menopause. Skeletal fragility has become part of what it means to be an older woman in Western culture. When the ice at White Creek Lodge broke my arm, I thought I would be blamed for not having looked after my bones properly, for having allowed deterioration and disintegration, so that disasters were just waiting to happen. In fact, American law doesn't allow flaky bones to be part of a legal counter-attack, but this didn't stop the White Creek Lodge's lawyer from trying hard to suggest that a back problem I'd had two years before the fracture meant that the condition of my bones was suspect. Had I had surgery for the back problem? Had I ever broken anything before? Or since? Was I, in other words, inherently crumbly?

In the 18th century, the popular search for sex differences found them everywhere, including in the skeleton.[1] Today, the experts have become much more precise about this, and the ageing female body is defined in terms of its bone mineral density, an exact figure derived from the interrogation of female bones, using dual energy X-ray absorptionetry screening machines. As Inge Klinge noted, when she studied the recent history of women's bones for her doctoral thesis, it's striking that this reduction to a brittle skeleton has arrived just at the time of women's emancipation to a fuller public life.[2]

The reduction of women to their bodies has a long history. In many systems of cultural thought, women *are* their bodies, whereas masculinity is something beyond and greater than the body – a propensity to rise above it, like angels or God. Minds capable of rational thought are accidental inhabitants of bodies; the masculinised self rescues the mind from its mundane corporeal location. Women's bodies, on the other hand, govern their selves in irrational and uncontrollable ways. Women have been hysterical walking wombs; polluters of the civil body; tiny, abnormally lateralised brains; genetic programmes for housework and childcare; now they're ropey skeletons as well. We can't trust our bodies in this very essence: the only structure that's left after death, when decay has disposed of the rest.

When Fuller Albright, a doctor in the USA, looked at 42 cases of fracture in 1941, his observation that 40 were women led him to invent the concept of 'postmenopausal osteoporosis'.[3] According to the *Oxford English Dictionary*, the term 'osteoporosis' comes from 'osteo' bone, and 'porosis' the condition of having 'minute interstices through which water, air, light, etc may pass'. Brittle bones, said Dr Albright, were caused by hormone deficiency. The menopause was by then already recognised medically as a 'deficiency' disease, a resounding example of system failure. Idle machines are the ultimate horror of a technological society. Only thus can we explain suggestions, made with utter seriousness, to the effect that all post-menopausal women might just as well get their breasts cut off, because this is the most efficient way to prevent breast cancer.[4] The redundant nature of post-menopausal breasts (and uteruses) stands for the obsolescence of older women themselves. Their bodies and lives are retired characters in a script that is best kept hidden from public view altogether.

When medicine labels a new condition, a recipe for its treatment isn't far behind. The condition of the menopause and its (nearly) inevitable consequence – osteoporosis – suggest that there's something about ageing in women that needs adjusting to prevent symptoms of decay. Enter the industry of hormone replacement therapy (HRT), which has led millions of women to be medicated with harmful drugs that have made pharmaceutical companies fortunes. By 2001, global sales of HRT amounted to $3.8 billion and 100 million women were taking it.[5] HRT successfully shifted the medical treatment of ageing women from psychology to gynaecology: women, constitutionally insanitised by their uteruses, could now be saved by the wonders of modern medicine. HRT is 'the ultimate case study in pharmaceutical marketing',[6] in how to make millions by inventing new conditions that need treatment, playing on people's susceptibilities, and ignoring the bad news about what drugs do to the body. HRT is an 'international tragedy' akin to thalidomide,[7] another drug prescribed for female instability, which caused thousands of babies to be born with limb and other defects. These disasters happen because the medicalised body is also a medicated one.

Yet you would never think that HRT's an international tragedy from the way in which the media and many intelligent people talk about the advisability of medicating ageing women's bodies. When a group of researchers looked at how the media reported three commonly used drugs (including one for osteoporosis), they found that 83% of news stories mentioned benefits and only 47% adverse effects. Forty one per cent of the stories cited experts or scientific studies with some financial link to companies making the drugs, but fewer than half disclosed this link.[8] Dr Robert Wilson's famous book *Forever feminine*, published in 1963, which attractively portrayed post-menopausal women as 'castrates' and argued the case for universal HRT, was paid for by the pharmaceutical company Wyeth, although this wasn't commonly known until recently. Wyeth holds 70% of the market in HRT, and its products have been among the fifty top selling drugs in the US for more than forty years.[9]

The use of hormones to treat the 'deficiency' disease of the menopause increased in the 1950s and 1960s, especially in the USA, where it was one of the top five prescribed drugs by the early 1970s. Not all countries went the same way: in the early 1990s, usage varied from less than 1% to 20%, with women in the USA being the most enthusiastic users, followed by women in the UK and Scandinavia, and those in continental Europe being much more cautious.[10] While doctors pushed the use of HRT to prevent disease, women have tended to take it for the short-term relief of menopausal symptoms,[11] mainly the hot flushes described by the French novelist George Sand in a letter to her editor in 1853: 'I experience the phenomenon of believing that I am sweating fifteen or twenty times a day and night...I have both the heat and the fatigue. I wipe my face with a white handkerchief and it is laughable because I am not sweating at all.'[12] In such narratives, the menopause features as temporary disablement: three quarters of women in English-speaking countries don't experience the menopause as troublesome.[13] They certainly don't use prevailing medical metaphors – 'declining' hormone production, 'decreasing' sensitivity of the hypothalamus to hormones, 'failing' ovaries – to describe it. What they want to talk about is other things: life after the menopause, new freedoms and possibilities.[14]

In the beginning, the medical arguments in favour of

universal HRT were simple: that the menopause is an unnatural event. Most women in the past would have died when they finished childbearing. (This is still true in some places in the world today.) The post-menopausal body is therefore a freak, and no-one should have to put up with it. Further support for this argument comes from the fact that post-menopausal women become significantly more like men with respect to heart disease and some cancers. 'Replacing' hormones should therefore abate this unwelcome move to gender equality: take this 'beautiful medication'[15] and all will be well.

The sad story of HRT is that it cannot offer this salvation. By the mid-1970s, it was clear that women who took the original formulation were *more*, not *less*, likely to develop risk factors for heart disease and other illnesses, especially cancer of the uterine lining, which was four to eight times more likely among HRT users.[16] Interestingly, this risk was known in the early medical research, which explored the possible protective health effects of artificial hormones for both men *and* women. The equivalent risk for men was prostate cancer: work on replacing men's hormones was consequently stopped. The risk of damage to women's uteruses, however, was evaluated differently.[17]

When the harmful effects of HRT began to emerge, the pharmaceutical industry responded, not by decreasing production, but by 'rehabilitating' HRT. First, they added another hormone, progesterone, to the oestrogen formula. Then they claimed that HRT had a new function altogether: protecting women's bones. Today, osteoporosis is defined as a major public health problem. In the UK alone, it's associated with 200,000 fractures a year.[18] Broken bones cost health care systems a lot to repair.

Medicating bodies to prevent the disaster of broken bones therefore makes economic sense. In 1994, the World Health Organization defined osteoporosis as a bone mineral density of 2.5 standard deviations or more below the mean value for healthy White women in their late twenties.[19]

A woman of my age (in her sixties) lives in a body which is the focus of institutionalised concern for many experts. We regularly receive 'invitations' to have our breasts squeezed between the blades of mammography machines, our uterine cervices scraped, and the state of our bones quantified. We have a lifetime of such offers, all made on the basis that we'll live longer and better with them than without them. But will we? Cancer experts say there's not enough evidence that the mammography business – currently worth $3-$4 billion a year in the USA – prevents breast cancer deaths.[20] Two female doctors who have headed such programmes and themselves developed breast cancer, despite being screened, have urged a fundamental rethink.[21] In the cervical cancer prevention industry, 1,000 women have to have cervical smear tests for thirty five years to prevent one death. During this period, one woman will also die despite being screened, and most of the 152 out of 1,000 whose smears yield 'abnormal' results will be anxious for no reason, since the majority of these abnormalities are minor and never become cancerous.[22]

The main function of medical screening isn't to prevent disease, but to change identities - to produce patients. 'Becoming a patient is not a trivial matter. It has profound health, social, psychological and economic consequences.'[23] Invitations to be screened ignore or make light of these consequences. For example, none of thirty one leaflets sent to women in seven countries about mammography screening mentioned any of the common harmful consequences of screening, such as anxiety, over-diagnosis and unnecessary surgery. Medical surveillance of the female body is presented as a form of liberation *from* the body.[24] Doctors are paid to get patients into screening programmes, and, until recently, consent forms for such tests in the UK had no space for patients to record an informed decision not to take part; all you could be was wilfully 'non-compliant'. Women imbibe the morality of the screening industry more readily than men. We are more law-abiding, accepting the logic of this industry which turns us into the police-people of our bodies, vigilantly searching for, and thus often finding, evidence of criminal activities. We overstate the benefits of screening by a factor of ten or more, and only a minority of us perceive it as causing harm.[25]

One aspect of this culturally embedded over-reading of screening's value in protecting our bodies is that men can feel excluded. In response, they demand parity by having access to screening for prostate cancer. When *The San Francisco Chronicle* published a piece about the manager of the city's baseball team who raved about the screening test for prostate cancer because it led him to have his own removed, two doctors who wrote to sound a note of evidence-based caution were compared with the Nazi doctor Joseph Mengele, and accused of having thousands of future deaths on their hands.[26] Like many such tests, the one for prostate cancer generates many diagnoses of problems which turn out to be false, while also missing established cancers.[27]

Having spotted the cultural deceit here, I'm a non-compliant patient, although I try to be pleasant at the same time. Before my fracture at the White Tee Lodge, I'd declined invitations to have bone mineral density screening because its overall effects are unknown, and because the programme is based on shaky logic. Most fractures are in women whose bones aren't thin, at least not as measured by the bone scanning devices that now form a routine part of the technology of health surveillance applied to women's bodies. Furthermore, one in six old age fractures is in men, and one in twelve men has osteoporosis.[28] Another reason for declining bone mineral density screening was that enough of me was being screened already. All this surveillance is such hard work. Then, after the fracture, I was afraid of the answer a test of my bone mineral density might give. What if the magic number was too low? How would this change my attitude to my body? What would I do about it?

Bone mineral density numbers are 'sexy': doctors believe they understand them, hospitals rely on them to generate income, and governments can cite them as measures of cost-conscious activity in fracture prevention.[29] Like much in medicine, the construction of 'abnormal' bone mineral density in postmenopausal women involved an arbitrary decision. It isn't that bones with a mineral density of less than 2.5 standard deviations below the mean, break, whereas those above this point don't, but that the association between bone mineral density and fracture risk must be constructed so as to justify medical intervention at some point. US doctors routinely intervene at a higher bone mineral density than UK doctors, prescribing drugs for women with thicker bones than their counterparts in the UK,[30] although there's nothing presumably in American women's bones to warrant this.

A friend of mine told me, with some seriousness and alarm, that she'd recently had her bones screened and had been informed that she had 'osteopenia'. This is a new condition, which hugely expands the number of women whose skeletons are at risk, and who therefore need preventive medication. Osteopenia is the infant cousin of osteoporosis, a state in which it is said that signs of possible future osteoporosis might begin to appear. The magic number here is a bone mineral density score between 1 and 2.5 standard deviations below the mean: any woman whose bones hit these figures has osteopenia, and is a candidate for preventive medication. Consequently, it's almost impossible for most women over fifty to be defined as normal. The World Health Organization criterion labels 30% of women over fifty as having osteoporosis and a much large proportion as suffering from its younger cousin.[31]

Underlying these shifts in medical labels and treatments are two models of women's bodies: the hormonal and the mineral. The HRT industry was built on the 'hormonal' body model: the notion that older women's bodies lack the hormonal profiles of younger women, that what is youthful must be normal, and that the proper response is to deceive the body into believing it's hormonally younger than it is. But the post-1970s rehabilitation of HRT proved to be only partial, and, as with many drugs, time and careful study revealed a battery of untoward effects, even with the addition of progesterone to 'oppose' the unwanted effects of artificial oestrogen. Women taking these newer formulations have significantly increased risks (compared with those not taking HRT) of heart disease, breast cancer, stroke, pulmonary embolism and incontinence.[32] The estimate in the USA is 1,400 extra cases of breast cancer; 1,200 of heart disease; and 1,400 of strokes a year on account of HRT.[33] These consequences, following on those of the original drugs, are why HRT has been dubbed an international tragedy.

With the evident failure of the hormonal body model, medical attention turned to the mineral version. The essential deficiency from which older women now suffer is no longer failing hormones, but flaky bones. The pre-eminence of the 'mineral' body has meant a whole new class of drugs – the biphosphonates – to prevent and treat osteoporosis/penia. These drugs are marketed directly for fracture reduction in postmenopausal women; global sales are around $2.7 million a year.[34] Biphosphonates have a very different mode of action from hormones. They alter the bones directly by decreasing the natural process of bone resorption. Since old bone is denser than new – it has less water and is more mineralised – the drug's effect on the formation of new bone appears to preserve bone mineral density. The biphosphonates are drugs that stay in the body for decades; there's no known method of removing them from the bones. As they prevent new bone from forming, they also inhibit the natural process of bone remodelling – the body's constant repair of microcracks in bones due to everyday activities. The overall effect may therefore well be to make bones *more*, not *less*, brittle. As with the hormonal answer to the problem of older women's bodies, it will take time for the true benefits and costs of these drugs to emerge, but the most recent evidence from the Fracture Intervention Trial in the USA suggests that the effect in conserving bone mineral density only lasts for five years, and there's no difference between medicated and unmedicated women in the ultimate endpoint, which is fractures.[35] Consistent with the theoretical observation that the drugs may increase bone brittleness, some doctors have also noted unusual fractures with delayed healing in treated women.[36]

The road sign introduced in the UK in 1981 warning of elderly or disabled pedestrians depicts the silhouette of a man using a cane leading a woman with the bent back characteristic of established osteoporosis. Old age is equated with vertebral collapse (her) and mobility aids (him). My own mother, she of the creaking knees, developed osteoporotic fractures in her seventies. She had sad tales to tell of tripping on uneven pavements and shattering vertebrae on the way to the shops. This counts as a risky 'family history'; like mother, like daughter, they say. But what is 'a family history'? Her mother, my maternal grandmother, died skeletally intact in her late eighties, with a back as straight as a board. Her daughter, my mother, was a heavy smoker all her life, had her first and only child in her forties, and was treated with steroids for another condition in her fifties. All these are associated with a greater propensity to break bones. In the epidemiology of bone fractures, genetic factors aren't actually a strong influence: the most important are one's propensity to fall, *how* one falls, 'protective neuromuscular responses' and the capacity of the body to absorb the energy produced by falling.[37] As a matter of well-concealed fact, 85% of fractures aren't explained by the decrease in bone density as women get older, and asking women questions about such factors as age, living circumstances and exercise is as good at predicting who will break their bones as the fancy bone densitometry machines.[38] The best protection against fracture isn't drugs, but exercise. Climbing stairs and walking fast are the most efficient ways to improve bone mineral density, and they have no known adverse effects (unless you fall, of course).[39] There's what the epidemiologists call a 'dose response' relationship here: the more the exercise, the stronger the bones. But the problem is that, unless like Laurie Taylor you join an expensive health club, exercise costs nothing, and pharmaceutical companies have nothing to gain from promoting it.

Two years ago, at the age of 61, I joined a classical ballet class. Now, twice a week, I stand at the barre with a group of lithe 20-year-olds who watch me with mixed amusement and horror. Some of them studiously avoid looking at me, and, when we have to choose partners to cavort across the studio floor, they look desperately round for younger companions. I feel like saying to them, old age isn't a disease, you know, and it certainly isn't contagious. You'll be old, too, one day. But, as the diarist May Sarton said, old age isn't interesting until you get there, and the surfeit of bodily experience that comes with age is a taboo subject.[40] The young talk about their bodies all the time, but the old, who might quite like to sometimes, must keep their mouths shut.

Old age is such a dismal subject, as Simone de Beauvoir discovered when she told people she was writing a book about it.[41] It's boring, like housework. Most of those who do housework are women, and old age is also a female speciality; in these respects, the lives of women are dismally invisible. In her book *Time on our side*, Dorothy Rowe talks of sitting on a train in England next to two young men who loudly discussed intimate details of their work, their expense accounts, etc for the whole of a long journey. The reason they made no concessions because of her presence was because they simply didn't notice it.[42]

Myself, I have learnt to play on the notion of eccentricity: this is one version of old age for women I can do something with. Older women don't have to obey the conventions of femininity any more. We don't have to watch people watching us because we no longer care what they think. As one old woman said to a social researcher, 'You can get away with all sorts of things when you're old because they think you're batty anyway'.[43]

Today, the problem of old age masks what it means to grow old. The cult of youthism merges easily with the overpowering policy statistics of the ageing population – what two sociologists have called 'apocalyptic demography'[44] – creating a nightmare of dependant pensioners, drains on health and welfare services, the detritus of a society in which earning money is the only mark of human value. Old people are an 'other', like immigrants, travellers, the disabled. In their book *I don't feel old*, Paul Thompson and his colleagues describe dominant stereotypes of ageing as follows: 'Old people think and move slowly. They are not creative and can't learn, change or grow. They dislike innovation and new ideas. They enter a second childhood and are egocentric. They become irritable and cantankerous, get shallow and enfeebled. They live in the past behind the times. Their minds wander and they reminisce. They are also often stricken with disease which restricts their movements. They have lost and cannot replace friends, spouses, jobs, status, power, influence and income. They have lost their desire and capacity for sex. Feeble, uninteresting, they await death, a burden to society, families, themselves.'[45]

It's even worse for women. 'The Wicked Old Witch, the Old Bad Mother, the Little Old Lady "cloud the individuality of every woman past 60".'[46] The Good Grandmother is the best available option here, but it can be a bit restrictive. Most of the grandmothers in children's books have grey hair, crabby faces, spectacles and sticks. They wear aprons, shawls and carpet slippers over ample pink flesh. Some have an eccentric verve for life; the granny in Arlene Alda's *Hurry, Granny Annie* (a favourite of mine for obvious reasons) rushes through the countryside at enormous speed chasing the sunset, garbed in striped bloomers, orange socks and trainers (though even she clutches a stick).[47] In Babette Cole's *The trouble with Gran*, Gran's embarrassing behaviour is due to the fact that she comes from another planet. Although she knits, accompanied by hat and teapot, she transports all the other 'OAPs' to her other planet, and then ends up running a travel agency in the family garage.[48] When children from thirty three countries were asked to draw their grandmothers for a competition in 1989-90, their depictions differed enormously. The most physically active grandmothers lived in India, the least in Western Europe. The Indian grandmothers were the most strongly integrated into society; in Switzerland, the Netherlands and most European countries, grandmothers hovered alone on the fringes of society with nothing very useful to do. Interestingly, and more hopefully, perhaps, grandmothers were typically depicted with some signs of ageing but garbed like teenagers: in one such drawing, a grandmother with a single remaining black tooth was roller skating wearing a bright pink mini skirt.[49]

Are we 'dentured crones' or 'leotarded achievers'?[50]

Or do we simply look in the mirror and dwell despondently on what we see? When I look in the mirror, I see a woman who is usually older than I feel (though on bad days the face looking back at me can be surprisingly young). This disjunction between age inside and age outside is a common feature of ageing. In her book, *Look me in the eye*, Barbara MacDonald describes seeing an old woman's body: '…I see my arm with the skin hanging loosely from my forearm and cannot believe that it is really my own. It seems disconnected from me; it is someone else's, it is the arm of an old woman. It is the arm of such old women as I myself have seen, sitting on benches in the sun with their hands folded in their laps; old women I have turned away from'.[51] Clara, aged 85, looks at a photo of herself: 'I see an old lady…I just brush it off. It isn't me'. [52] It's an identity-survival trick: I don't like what I see, so it isn't me. The person in the mirror is a stranger, and the question one asks is not unlike the experience of conjoined twins separated by surgery: Can I have become a different person while I still remain myself? [53]

In her *The last gift of time: Life after sixty*, Carolyn Heilbrun recounts how she saw herself in a hotel mirror one day and gave up wearing dresses on the spot.[54] Mirrors are prominent in accounts of ageing, because you have to see the older body to know it's yours. The mirror isn't a device for uncovering objective truth, but a method of seeing how others see us. That's why women look in them more than men; as a social minority group, we must study both ourselves and the way the majority group see us. Getting old *is* a profoundly gendered experience; women have to ward off the signs of ageing far more than men. Many dye their hair; choose clothes to conceal sagging bodies; buy expensive cosmetic alterations; constantly watch their weight; and generally pretend to be sweet and sprightly, when what they feel most of the time is something quite different.

Virginia Woolf knew that, objectively, ageing is nonsense: '…some we know to be dead though they walk among us,' she wrote sagely in her playful novel about gender, *Orlando*. 'Some are not yet born though they go through the forms of life; others are hundreds of years old though they call themselves thirty six. The true length of a person's life …is always a matter of dispute.'[55] While a disease-free old age is unrealistic for many, until 85 there's a greater then even probability of no disability or ill health.[56] But the visual stereotype of an older body makes the body an unwelcome guest in the universe of the self – or like an 'involuntary change of dress'.[57] Ageing, like illness, is primarily an experience of embodiment: a time in our lives when it's hard to pretend that we are in any sense separate from our bodies. The body is against us, declared Yeats at 57, blind in one eye and fearing deafness: 'Being old makes me tired and furious; I am everything that I was and indeed more, but an enemy has bound and twisted me so that although I can make plans and think better than ever, I can no longer carry out what I plan and think'.[58] The old live in, and with, time, in a way that the young don't have to. Death is 'the one concept you can't deconstruct' learns Morris Zapp in David Lodge's novel *Small world*; captured by terrorists, he suddenly finds he loses his enthusiasm for post-modernism.[59]

The young can be profoundly disparaging about the old. In *The loneliness of the dying*, Norbert Elias writes about himself as a young man attending a lecture in

Cambridge by a famous physiologist. The lecturer came into the lecture hall, shuffling slowly, dragging his feet. 'I caught myself wondering, why does he drag his feet like that? Why can he not walk like a normal human being? I at once corrected myself. He can't help it, I told myself. He is very old.'[60] The young simply have no basis in their experience for imagining how it feels when the self tells the body to move, and the body resists because the muscles have hardened, the joints are stiff and the bones grate against one another. Because the old are caricatures of the young, the young must laugh at the old in order to break the connection.

Most of my own sense of being old(er) has nothing to do with present body experiences. It's about simply having lived quite a long time. I'm aware of my body's history, and also of my own. 'In old age, embodied knowledge represents the accumulation of a lifetime of self-understanding. Embodied knowledge encompasses people's historical experience of their bodies.'[61] Wrinkles, for example, are the result of facial activity. The more you smile and frown, and weep and laugh, the more your face is a map of all you've been through. In this accretion of memories, lessons learnt, traps fallen into, pleasures had and miseries survived, I feel I have acquired a little of something I hesitantly call 'wisdom'. It's this feature of ageing, combined with their roles as domestic angels, that explains why 'sober, ancient' women have traditionally been charged with various important community activities. 'From lying in to laying out, older women were the best guides to the body,' writes Laura Gowing in her history of women, touch and power in 17th century England.[62] This is also why science fiction writer Ursula LeGuin would pick an old woman, over sixty, from behind the costume jewellery counter of the local Woolworths or the betel-nut booth in the village marketplace, to represent planet earth on a spaceship from another galaxy. The old woman's hair has faded, her skin's not dewy fresh, and sometimes her feet hurt a lot, but only old women like her have 'experienced, accepted and acted the entire human condition'.[63]

While we wait for our chance on the spaceship, we can cheer ourselves up with the news that we'd do well to spend our declining years on another kind of ship. Cruses to the Caribbean are cheaper for us and society than what are euphemistically called 'assisted living facilities'. [64] The scenery's better, and so is the health care. Perhaps there are also fewer opportunities to break our bones.

8

Two in one

ori and Reba Schappell are sisters, living together
in the same US town, but they never go shopping
together because Reba likes shopping efficiently
with a list, while Lori browses and impulse buys.[1] There's
nothing extraordinary about such differences between
members of the same family. What's out-of-the-ordinary
here is that Lori and Reba are conjoined twins. They're
joined at the head: one body flows without boundaries
into the other. Going shopping separately therefore calls
for more than the usual sisterly techniques of agreeing
to spend time apart. If Reba goes shopping with her list,
Lori is there but not there: she chooses to ignore what
the body joined to hers is doing. But what or who is it in
this case that isn't there?

Conjoined twins are objects of significant media
interest today. In the past, they often starred in 'freak'
shows. Chang and Eng Bunker, the original 'Siamese'
twins, were born in Siam (Thailand) in 1811, joined by a
band of flesh five inches long and nine inches thick. They
spent their adult lives farming in the US, where they
fathered ten and twelve children respectively, maintaining
two families a mile apart and taking it in turns to live in
each other's houses. Like many unseparated twins, they

were experts at teamwork, and had no trouble with the concept of two identities sharing the same bodily space, although other people did, particularly with the notion of shared sexual intimacy.[2]

It's rare for conjoined twins to request separation.[3] They don't, it seems, usually feel trapped by their bodily configuration – conjoinment is part of their concept of themselves. This is especially so when there are areas of common tactile sensation, and where both have the ability to move shared limbs. Proprioceptive feedback of the same body in space happens in the brains of both twins. Each brain holds a map of the shared body, and this is part of each twin's body image and physical individuality. The Tocci brothers, for example, born in 1878, each had his own arms, but a single body (abdomen, anus, penis and two legs, each controlled by one twin).[4]

Such bodies/people ill fit our notions of bounded individuality. Three reactions are possible: (i) one twin is simply extra flesh attached to the other; (ii) they're two psychologically separate individuals who happen to share a body; and (iii) they're accidentally and cruelly joined and should therefore be separated if possible.[5] The second view is the only one that really fits the facts of how conjoined twins live together, but it's the last that takes precedence in their medical treatment. Surgical separation forces twins apart, into a pretence of normally bounded individuals. Since there's usually a shortage of body parts to go round, neither twin can actually ever be 'normal'; but at least there's no affront to conventional sensibility any more.

Hippocrates referred to 'pathographies' as having the power to reveal the hidden structures of body and mind.[6] What is a person? Someone who is liveborn, with a functioning brain capable of sustaining an existence independently of her/his mother.[7] Giuseppina Santina Foglia, separated from her twin, Maria, at the age of six, asked after the surgery, 'Is it really me? Am I really Myself?'. Katie and Eilish Holton were joined shoulder to pelvis with two legs between them; when they were three and a half years old, doctors sculpted them into two separate bodies. Katie died, and afterwards Eilish would look to her side where Katie had been and cry; when given an artificial leg, she called it 'Katie'.[8]

The notion of 'unjust embodiment'[9] – being locked in, rather than simply sharing, a body or parts of one – comes from a culture obsessed with the idea that you can't be a person without a body of your own. The fascination provoked by conjoined twins derives, not from their rarity – one in 50,000 to one in 200,000 births – but from the challenge they pose to this sacred cultural canon. 'FREE AT LAST' screamed a newspaper headline when twins Carmen and Rosa Taveras were surgically separated in 1993.[10] We hail this as one of the miracles of modern medicine: to liberate people from a bodily entanglement which is a mere accident of birth, a prison from which they must surely want most desperately to escape. Law and medicine operate with the same paradigm: adjusting the bodily defect of conjoined twins is part of a much larger cultural enterprise in which citizenship includes bodily 'normalisation' as a right and a duty. We must aspire to a certain kind of body: a standard body with all its limbs, one that doesn't cause offence, which has no unwelcome protrusions or effluences, and no unexpected openings or closures. The 'normal' healthy body is a moral obligation supported by the weight of law, and made possible by miraculous medical intervention.

Consider the strange history of false teeth.[11] In the nineteenth century, these were disapproved of as vanity: one should make do with the teeth one had, with the natural rate of decay and loss. Anyway, artificial replacements were limited and useless. Queen Elizabeth 1 resorted to stuffing her cheeks with cloth, and George Washington tried to keep his mouth firmly shut. The history of the world has been considerably shaped by dental problems: Washington, for example, suffered much during the Revolutionary War, and Queen Elizabeth was in the company of other monarchs, such as Gustavus Vasa of Sweden and Louis XIV of France, in taking wild decisions while in dental agony. By the 18th century, you could order dentures by mail; these were populated by teeth extracted from dead soldiers, graveyards or the mouths of the poor, who sold them for food they then couldn't eat. These mail order dentures were ornamental and didn't help their new owners to eat, either – they had to be removed at the dinner table!

When the National Health Service arrived in Britain in 1946, its main impact in the early days was the democratisation of false teeth. Are false teeth part of the body? Such questions proliferate with the growing industry of organ transplants: kidneys, livers, lungs, hearts, faces, hands; each of us could theoretically be composed of many bodies. It's hard to dispose of the notion that, in incorporating bits of other people's bodies into our own, we are also absorbing their identities. The notion that receiving someone else's blood is to accept their essence runs through the history of blood transfusion.[12] Perhaps the self's expression in bodily organs applies most of all,

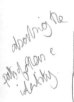

in Western culture, to the heart, which is linked to the soul as the central repository of human identity, although other cultures locate the soul in different places. For us, the heart is the site of emotion, the place where feelings are stored, from which love comes. If we are given someone else's heart, is it possible that we inherit their emotional, as well as their physical, existence?

This is, in part, the logic of cannibalism. The Bimim-Kuskusmin of New Guinea eat their dead to ensure that the dead's knowledge and power are not lost, but incorporated into the living clan; the still fertile wife of a dead man is supposed to eat bits of his penis to ensure her ability to have more children.[13] Cannibalism, 'the last taboo', has a long, distressing history about both the motive and consequences of incorporation, and about how ordinary human beings can be driven to extreme behaviour in the interests of preserving their bodies.[14]

One way to see the modern manufacture of the body is to understand that we're all becoming cyborgs: hybrids of technology and biology. Our bodies regularly incorporate non-human material – metals, ceramics, polymers – as well as bits of other bodies. We host amalgam, porcelain and gold embellishments in our mouths; have our eyesight saved with synthetic lenses; use mechanical pacemakers and synthetic valves to regulate our hearts; incorporate artificial hips and knees; and accept pins, staples and sutures of every kind.[15] We can have our breasts chopped off and replaced, or reduced or expanded with synthetic substances; our faces rearranged; kilos of flesh lifted from our stomachs and our buttocks; false or adjusted sexual organs; and a whole array of prosthetic limbs await, gendered to fit standards of masculinity and femininity, just like us.[16] The aesthetic paradigm that drives the prosthetic industry is masculine: women sewed their own breast prostheses until well into the 1970s.[17] Prosthetic limbs owe their main development to the grim accidents in the mills and factors of 19th century capitalism,[18] and then to the legacy of more overt war: giving soldiers with severed or damaged limbs new arms and legs to call their own.[19] The use of biomaterials in human bodies goes back a long way, to the ancient Chinese and the Aztecs, and the surgical sages of India and beyond.[20] Today, the commodification of body parts has reached new heights with the globalisation of a 'human body shop'.[21] Large corporations obtain, store and redistribute human tissue in a multimillion dollar industry. The rhetoric of altruism – the 'gift' of life – conceals a trade in commercialised body parts underscored by the 'open secret' of a black market, in which bodies in the developing world supply kidneys and other organs to bodies in the West.[22]

Cosmetic surgery – 'competitive working on the self'[23] – has now entered the realm of the everyday, and popular magazines admonish the ageing and the subjectively blemished to buy improvements, just as they would a new kitchen or a sofa in place of the one that sags, because its springs have long gone. The first recorded use of cosmetic surgery to 'improve' the ageing body was on a Polish aristocrat in the early 1900s, who designed her own facelift.[24] That's how this form of surgery began: as a sculpting of the face, and especially of the nose, regarded as a prominent bodily sign of character, and notably of racial identity. Celebrity culture, psychoanalysis and cosmetic surgery all became growth industries at about the same time, and all offered a spectacularly gendered view of the body as a plastic product.[25] By 1996, there was one episode of 'aesthetic' surgery for every 150 Americans, 89% on women, with breasts, thighs, buttocks and tummies the favoured targets (the male equivalents were breast reduction, hair transplants and nose jobs).[26]

Cosmetic surgery is about the imagined body; it's about our culturally induced fantasies of ourselves: 'The body is nothing until it's jolted into being the image of something it could become...'[27] The 'postmodern' body is a fantasy of 'rearranging, transforming and correcting, limitless improvement and change'.[28] These new plastic bodies are final proof that the human body is a cultural product. In this, our bodies share their fate with us: both bodies and selves are moulded by the environment – by cultural values and expectations; through prescriptions and proscriptions; and by means of vanities, crimes, fables and foibles of every possible kind.

the human body as a cultural product

Conjoined twins are one of three human conditions which challenge the one brain/identity-one body philosophical tradition of Western thought. The other two are pregnancy and breastfeeding. In the 1970s, two US researchers, one dressed as a pregnant woman, the other holding a large cardboard box in front of her, rode up and down elevators in a New Haven apartment building to observe people's reactions. Those who entered the elevator shunned the pregnant researcher by standing well away from her, and this reaction was more marked in men.[29] Pregnancy, the researchers concluded, is a social stigma. All types of stigma – physical deformities, character blemishes (inferred through mental illness or imprisonment, for example) and the 'tribal' stigmas – of ethnicity, nationality or religion – are 'undesired differentness'. The person with the stigma becomes that

How did they know she was being shunned rather than cared for?

stigma in the eyes of others, who consequently turn away from something which isn't quite human.[30]

The stigma of pregnancy is, of course, odd, since most of the people in the world are women, and most of them are pregnant at least once. But the pregnant female body isn't the norm, the standard against which all bodies are judged. Pregnancy disturbs because it disrupts dualistic thinking. In the body of a pregnant woman, there is at least one other body, and the point of its emergence is the most extreme splitting of one into two. What, then, is the 'self' here? Pregnancy is subjectively a condition of ambiguity. What am I growing inside myself, and who am I, now that this is happening? Such feelings are intensified when the fetus is known to be male,[31] for here a condition of 'not-me' inside me clearly obtains. In other ways, pregnant and postnatal bodies constantly threaten to break boundaries because they're disturbingly non-stable entities: leaking and seepage are routine, uncontrollable events.[32] The breasts eject colostrum and milk; glandular discharges, amniotic fluid and blood escape the vagina; and the vomiting of early pregnancy and labour takes women by surprise. Anxiety, mood swings and hysteria – marks of femininity in general – are exacerbated in and after pregnancy, making the easy flow of tears another unwelcome effluent. The fetus within swells its mother's abdomen and breasts, and these changed contours affect not only how pregnant women think of themselves, but their relationship with the material world: 'In pregnancy I literally do not have a firm sense of where my body ends and the world begins. My automatic body habits become dislodged; the continuity between my customary body and my body at this moment is broken.'[33] Due to these unstable, negatively viewed relationships between body and environment, pregnant women withdraw from public space. Pregnancy is a form of agoraphobia: the disruption of the usual barriers between internal and external space act to confine women to the private space of the home.[34]

People touch the stomachs of pregnant women with horror and fascination, and often without asking permission, as though the condition of pregnancy suspends women's right to bodily privacy – which it does. In the West, we're now living in the midst of an epidemic of state-sanctioned assault on the bodies of childbearing women. The use of force has been associated with the rise of obstetricians as the masters of childbirth ever since the first crude forceps were used to drag babies out in the 18th century. Today, obstetricians just cut women's abdomens and uteruses open, and yank the baby out. In many places today, Caesarean section is well on the way to becoming what usually happens.[35] The splitting of one body into two, the most disturbing drama of all for a culture centred on the one body / one identity doctrine, is rationalised by becoming yet another wonderful medical accomplishment. This is the other curious aspect of the stigma of pregnancy: that, without pregnancy, human bodies wouldn't exist at all. Science and medicine would have turned procreation into a technological process if they could have done, but a uterus inside a female body remains a necessary incubator for the unborn child, even one conceived in a petri dish. Human society can't do without women's bodies, although it's certainly tried, which is perhaps one reason why it does so much to them.

Pamela Rae Stewart was the first pregnant women to be charged in the USA under the new regime of fetal rights protection. The charge, in 1987, was criminal neglect of a child, because Pamela was reluctant to follow medical advice. Many other such crimes have been concocted since, including that of exposing the fetus to alcohol, tobacco and other drugs (delivering controlled substances to minors via the umbilical cord, as though the uterus is some sort of unlicensed public house), and 'vehicular homicide' – car accidents resulting in miscarriage.[36] The rights of the fetus are used to justify court-ordered obstetrical interventions, and these are contributing to the rise in surgical childbirth. Most such court orders in the USA are used for poor, minority ethnic women, who are least able to assert their rights against the state's promulgation of a war against them.[37] Like the populations of the nineteen countries the USA has invaded since 1945, this is an undemocratic war, lacking the assent of those on whose behalf it's purportedly being fought. Mothers go to prison for their supposed anti-fetal sins; state 'protection' of fetal rights is at the cost of women's autonomy. But, in male-dominated cultures, women's right to bodily integrity has always been conditional, so this is really only a new version of an old oppression.

Myths need strategies to sustain them; in order to exert their power, they must resonate with the 'set' of a culture. Ultrasound imaging of the fetus was originally developed in the 1970s to distinguish between pregnancy and other abdominal tumours.[38] For an ultrasound examination, the woman lies down so the technician can access the fetus within her. Her abdomen is oiled, and the scanning device moved across it. The fetal image is projected on the screen so that the technician, the obstetrician, and often the father as well, can see it. As one doctor said, fetuses couldn't be taken seriously so long as they were recluses in opaque wombs; only what can be seen can be believed.[39] Ultrasound has turned pregnancy into a 'good show',[40] starring the fetus as an apparently autonomous acrobat in the theatre of the mother's womb, with her role as producer a forgotten byline.[41] In the two-dimensional, cross-sectional displays on ultrasound VDUs, the fetus floats in free space, and the maternal body is eclipsed from view. The impact of the poised, separate fetal image is much like that of the first pictures of planet earth provided by 'man's' exploration of space. Then the magic blue-green orb impressed us with its vulnerability: there it hangs, all on its own, subject to the whims and fancies of the entire universe. It needs protection, just as fetuses on ultrasound screens move us with their vitality and fragility to construct this ogre of the selfish maternal body.

Breastfeeding is the third paradoxical condition which challenges our normal assumption of one body / one identity. The breastfeeding child's body is dependent for survival on the mother's, and the mother needs the child to relieve the discomfort of milk-full breasts. The two are separate but attached, in another out-of-the-ordinary state of mutual dependence. Breastfeeding isn't 'extra' ordinary, but just not ordinary, where 'ordinary' means total body separation.[42] The reason breastfeeding offends isn't because it reveals the female breast: tabloids and porn magazines do that all the time. Breastfeeding is offensive in suggesting that different bodies are biologically tied to one another, and that parts of women's bodies are regularly used by children rather than by men in some kind of antediluvian and unnecessary ('irrational'?) resistance to modern technology. Significantly, women often don't

regard their newborn babies as entirely separate beings.[43]
This is a reaction which has provided much material for a
psychoanalytic industry built on the precepts of masculine
psychology, with its stern insistence on the morality of the
independent self.

Norms of male embodiment accommodate pregnancy
and childbirth badly – so badly that both are defined as
forms of illness in anti-discrimination and equal
opportunity legislation.[44] But the real illness here is the
offence that fusion of bodily boundaries creates: because
we *are* our bodies, we must *have* bodies of our own. The
mutual dependence of bodies is tolerated only in
heterosexual eroticism, and then fleetingly: to be
permanently joined to another is a malady. In this cultural
script, women's bodily ambiguity puts them aside. They
are 'morphologically dubious': 'If we define the monster
as a bodily entity that is anomalous and deviant vis-à-
vis the norm, then we can argue that the female body
shares with the monster the privilege of bringing out a
unique blend of fascination and horror.'[45] What would
it do to our ideas about bodies and selves if the normal
human body were female and pregnant, and then joined
to another through lactation; and if every other kind of
body was seen as a curious departure from this?

The law of uncivil actions

Three and a half years after the accident at White Creek Lodge, I sit on the floor of my living room in London surrounded by files and papers sprouting multicoloured post-it notes. Holding up my right hand, I promise 'to tell the truth, the whole truth and nothing but the truth'. The room is empty, but only afterwards do I realise the absurdity of the right-hand gesture.

I am very nervous. This is an episode in the long drawn out case of *Oakley v White Creek Lodge*. The case is about the law relating to accidental injury, but it's also about how bodies feature in legal systems: our conditional right to live in an intact body. 'Have you ever been a plaintiff in a lawsuit before today?' asks the White Creek Lodge's lawyer, sitting by his conference call phone in Denver. 'Have you ever been convicted of any crimes?' No, but it certainly feels like a criminal mistake to have been dragged into the pathological 'baroque complexity'[1] of the American legal system. The 'compensation culture' – 'suing the living daylights out of those we blame for our misfortunes'[2] – rests on the essential lie of capitalism: that money equals happiness. The most important human rights are those to property and wealth; contentiousness in the pursuit of these rights has become one hallmark of a good citizen.

The US litigation industry is infamous; being a lawyer is recognised as a route to a comfortably, if not fabulously, wealthy life. The US spends five times more of its GNP than its major industrial competitors on personal injury cases.[3] When 81-year-old Stella Liebeck sued McDonalds for millions of dollars after spilling a cup of coffee on herself, she gave her name to an annual award for the most ridiculous US lawsuit. The winner of the 2006 Stella Award was a Mr Merv Grazinski from Oklahoma City, who reputedly bought a thirty-two foot Winnebago motor home, set the cruise control to seventy miles per hour during his first trip with it on the freeway, and went in the back to make himself a sandwich. The vehicle crashed and overturned, and Mr Grazinski sued the manufacturers for not saying in the handbook you couldn't do this. He won $1,750,000 and a new motor home.[4]

The three occupational groups that have increased most in the US over the last thirty years are lawyers, computer programmers and prisoners.[5] Lawyers flourish in the USA for two main reasons: the welfare system leaves many holes that injury compensation can fill; and legal practice was deregulated in the 1970s, so that, for the first time, lawyers were able to advertise their services and tout for business. The critical moment in the story of the US litigation explosion was the verdict of Justice Harry Blackmun in 1977 in the case of a Phoenix law firm which advertised its services in the local paper. The State's legal association tried unsuccessfully to discipline the firm; the case then went to the Supreme Court, where Justice Blackmun, famous for his previous upholding of women's right to abortion, declared that the constitution protects lawyers' rights to advertise.[6] Before this point, going to law was regarded as a necessary evil, and even lawyers themselves took the view that it was their moral duty not to solicit custom and stir up grievance for profit. In a standard legal treatise of 1853, the particular legal habit of ambulance-chasing which initiated my own case against White Creek Lodge was described as 'so well-known and so obviously improper as to require no extensive comment'.[7] It happened, and lawyers could be jailed for it. One had only to consider the parallels with medicine to grasp the inequity of the practice, for if doctors persuaded people to be ill so they could make money out of treating them, who would benefit? (Some people, of course, would say this is exactly what does happen in some areas of health care today.)

Following the Blackmun verdict, other decisions allowed lawyers to solicit the business of 'persons known to have legal interests', at first by mail and then in person. This isn't just a question of lawyers visiting the bedsides of women with fractured limbs, but of their guaranteed presence at all natural and unnatural disasters, from ferryboat sinkings and mine cave-ins to aeroplane crashes. In 1987, after one of these events, a lawyer's 'runner' reportedly dressed as a priest to gain the confidence of grieving families. When the roof of a store collapsed in Texas, representatives of a local law firm posed as Red Cross workers, digging out victims so as to turn them into clients.[8]

My lawyer, Larry Barnard, was notified by the surgeon who fixed my fracture that here was a potentially profitable case for him. I don't recall the surgeon asking me first whether he could disclose confidential information about me to someone else. Larry works with eleven others in an office I've never visited, not far from the hospital to which he chased me on that icy day in December 2000. The firm specialises in medical malpractice, personal injury cases and product liability law – the biggest money-earners. 'This could be a million dollar case,' enthuses Larry at the beginning of our legal saga. Whom is he trying to persuade? The agreement I signed with him was on a no-win, no-fee basis – the so-called 'contingency fee' practice which is the 'Big Rock Candy Mountain' of contemporary US law,[9] making more overnight millionaires than just about any other business.[10] If he loses the case, I don't pay and he doesn't earn. If he wins, I pay the costs of pursuing it and he takes a share of any remaining proceeds. 'Winning' here is significantly termed 'recovery' – the illness of becoming a litigant will finally be over.

The contingency fee industry is openly run for profit, which means it operates according to the profiteer's own rules and timescale for the largest cash awards possible. Sometimes, if the lawyer has cashflow problems, the rush is on to get a quick settlement, but otherwise it's in the lawyer's interest to let the case run on. The average case takes six years to reach a trial.[11] Since he (it's usually a 'he') is fronting the money, it's *his* action not yours. Again, consider what would happen if doctors practised on this basis. With a financial interest in the outcome of treatment, they would profit from turning transient ailments into serious conditions, and from giving treatments that cause further financially profitable illnesses. It's for this reason that, in most countries, doctors and lawyers are prohibited from having a direct financial stake in what happens to their clients.

A 'good injury case' is a plum for the contingency fee lawyer. My own plum proceeds on a very relaxed schedule; the Barnard lawyers clearly have no cashflow problem. It takes seventeen months to settle the agreement between us, and then two years to draft what is called in legalese 'the Complaint' – my case against White Creek Lodge. In Civil Action no 4DB-09-1648-03VN, I become the Plaintiff, and accuse White Creek Lodge of 'gross, reckless, careless, indifferent and negligent conduct', allowing the path on which I fell to be in a dangerous and unsafe condition due to the accumulation of ice and/or snow. The result, says the Complaint document, is 'serious bodily injuries', some or all of which may be permanent. These injuries have necessitated costly medical treatment and painful physical rehabilitation, and have caused 'great physical pain and suffering, mental anguish, discomfort, inconvenience, distress, embarrassment, humiliation and loss of the ability to enjoy the pleasures of life' as well as an ability to perform my usual 'material acts and duties'. To make up for all these losses, I demand judgement against White Creek Lodge for an amount in excess of $175,000, plus the costs of the case.

The black and white text of the Complaint document impresses on me that, unlike the TV soap operas which celebrate the cultural ideal of American law, this case is now really happening. I didn't write the Complaint, nor did the lawyer consult me on what he should say in it. This sense I have of playing a part that somebody else has written in my own life is confirmed in the original version of the Complaint, which included my ex-husband and asked for a further $175,000 for the loss to him of my 'services, companionship, support, assistance, society, comfort, happiness and consortium'; because he has to pay all *my* medical costs; and because *he* will suffer from *my* loss of earnings and earning capacity. A few emails erase Plaintiff-Husband from the complaint, but I remain astounded by the sexist ideology (and by the possibility that I might have won twice as much if I'd played along with it).

Personal injury cases are 'the heart and soul'[12] of tort law – the law of 'civil wrongs' that decides when people should be financially compensated for adverse events that happen to their bodies or their minds. In medieval times, if someone was injured by the direct actions of another, he or she was automatically entitled to damages. It was the burgeoning entrepreneurial activity of the Industrial Revolution that introduced into tort law the obligation to *prove* wrongdoing. New railways and factories made injuries to the body caused by machines a major social problem. The industrialists wanted to protect themselves from this financial liability, so the onus was put on injured workers to prove wanton negligence. Today in the US, most civil cases considered by juries involve bodily injury claims.[13]

Preceding the fiction of 'recovery' in modern tort law is something called 'discovery' – the process of gathering together documents and other evidence before taking a case forward. 'Discovery' involves 'agonizingly detailed evaluation of the unevaluable'[14] for all aspects of the case: pain, mental anguish; medical and rehabilitation costs; disability; loss of employment and earnings; and every other kind of loss the injured person may be said to have suffered. The textbooks are explicit about what lawyers have a right to probe into: all details of health care; all current symptoms and any prognoses given; effects on employment and earnings, present and future; and impact on 'social life, sex life, sporting activities, hobbies, housework, DIY and so on'.[15]

In the interests of 'discovery', I sign a form (with my left hand) authorising release of my medical records. The hospital in Colorado sends copies to my lawyer, and he forwards them to me. The same thing happens with the hospital in London and my long-suffering GP. The result is a heavy parcel of 339 photocopied pages of incidents in the life of my body, and other people's interpretations of these, expensively transported to Denver and then back to North London. Thankfully, the first eleven years of my life are missing. I had forgotten the onychocryptosis (ingrown toenail) of my right first toe, but not the plantar wart I had gouged out of my left foot in 1956. What purpose do these details serve? When it comes to more recent stuff about cervical smears and stress at work, I am embarrassed and upset to think of these items lying around in legal offices thousands of miles away for any prying eyes to see.

When novelist Nina Bawden was injured and saw her husband die in a horrific train derailment in North London in May 2002, she described getting compensation as 'an obstacle race' in which 'evidence of continuing damage has to be proved by expensive medical specialists who are employed by the lawyers to read and report upon almost all a victim's medical history'. In her case, this included the irrelevance of a broken wrist sustained while cycling down a Shropshire lane on the night of her eighteenth birthday. In such cases, the lawyers, Bawden notes, seemingly have the right to interrogate one's whole life: 'both physical and emotional:

my earnings as a writer, my banking history, my shopping and eating habits...'[16]

When I said I consented to release of my medical records, I meant the records relevant to this case. I didn't mean the entire medical history of my body. They didn't tell me that 'discovery' means invasion of privacy.[17] They didn't mention this sense you get of being held morally responsible for every sickness or purported sickness inscribed in what is necessarily only a very partial record of your body's life on planet earth. What is the 'endogenous depression' which caused my body not to sleep back in 1990? I thought I said the problem was a sex discrimination case at work. I once had one of those DNA ('did not attend') letters from a hospital. and I had to write back pointing out that I did, but they got the date wrong. My letter isn't in the records, so only the hospital's stands, proving my (apparent) unreliability. Why does my gynaecologist keep writing to my GP, puzzled about my refusal to let the mineral density of my bones be examined? I thought I told him I wouldn't want to take the drugs he'd prescribe if the results were on the 'bad' side of the magic numbers doctors have devoted to labelling women's skeletons. In the US hospital notes, my weight is recorded as 233 pounds, but morbid obesity isn't one of my moral failings – someone wrote a '2' instead of a '1'. In letters from the London fracture clinic to my GP, I have several years deducted from my age, and am said (incorrectly) to be a sociologist working for the hospital and writing textbooks for medical students. Moreover, I have reputedly fractured my *left* arm. No wonder some patients have the wrong bits of their bodies removed.

The point is that the 'evidence' the lawyers have

discovered is the text of these partial and erroneous records. I stare at the 339 pages and wonder what to do with them. In the end, I feel obliged to read every word, because (I suppose) that's what Larry Barnard and his colleagues are doing in their smart offices in Denver, and I don't want them to know things about me that I don't. Besides, there's always a chance I might learn something useful about my body from these notes. I do certainly pick up more about my post-fracture problems than any of the doctors I saw told me, which I find interesting. 'I assume it must be a neuropraxia,' wrote a doctor at the London fracture clinic three months after the accident. 'The lesion must be a degenerative one, there is virtually complete loss of function within all modalities including sympathetic function,' declared the nerve specialist. Then comes the astonishing, '...her fracture is united and no further treatment is required', followed eighteen months post-accident by the bald, deceitful statement 'Recovery will be complete'.

Well, I knew they decided not to see me any more because the fact that I couldn't feel my hand wasn't their business, but I did keep telling them that, so why isn't it recorded in the notes? The absence of this information hardly helps Larry Barnard represent my case accurately to the White Creek Lodge's lawyers. One form of 'recovery'– the attributed medical one – is obstructing the other – the 'recovery' of money to compensate for (as if anything could) what's happened. Only the naïve, and I was certainly one of them at the beginning of all this, would suppose that lawyers are interested in the truth, and that an important part of the truth is the victim's perspective. The 'protection' of the law doesn't work like that. It exposes you, raw and bleeding and misrepresented, to vultures whose only interest is in turning your bodily damage into a source of income for themselves. There's no single moment when I realise this; it grows on me slowly, like a new illness.

My US lawyer isn't good at communicating. He doesn't reply to emails, letters or faxes, and phone calls to his office yield the usual vapid American guffaw at my name ('Ann(ie) Oakley'), and the unprofessional response that they don't know where Mr Barnard is. I don't think they know where London is, either, or (I fear) any country outside their own. The farcical nature of our 'communication' reaches its height when Larry Barnard gets his PA to email me, demanding to speak to me at a time when I can't, because I'm teaching. My email reply never reaches him because there's now some bug in his email system which blocks all my emails (is the bug, I wonder, responding to the eponymous 'Ann(ie) Oakley'?). Then an email asks me to phone him at home, which I do, only to get a recorded message informing me that this number is blocked to unrecognised callers.

As all this drives me to desperation, I suggest Larry Barnard might like to give the case to someone else. For a while, then, he swings into action, asking me questions he's asked and I've answered before: how much pain do I have? Can I provide a 'status' of my current medical condition? How much time did I have off work? What is my wage loss situation? Can I remember if it was snowing when I fell? Do I have the addresses of the colleagues who were with me? This is not a case to which he gives much time; it enters his consciousness only when I, or the 'due process' of the law, force it to.

A month after White Creek Lodge is served with my Complaint, the local judge orders a 'case management conference', whose date is then changed twice for unknown reasons, but this is for the lawyers, not me. It acquires a helpful urgency when, after a further month, the insurers of White Creek Lodge go bankrupt. This dashes Larry Barnard's hopes of making a small fortune out of me, and it suggests to me that we should stop the whole thing. But there's no easy stopping with a contingency fee agreement; if we do, I must pay all the costs so far. From then on, the saga degenerates further: more failed communications; dates announced and cancelled; obscure juridical decrees; and general confusion about whose case this is, and why it's happening – it isn't mine, for sure.

Tort cases in the USA are decided by juries, although few cases ever get as far as a trial.[18] It had never entered my head when I embarked on this sorry journey that I'd be expected to stand in a Colorado court over a period of possibly several weeks in front of unsympathetic lawyers and a jury of unknown attitude in order to support my claim that my brief sojourn at White Creek Lodge has damaged my body, my identity and my life. The case is first set for jury trial on 4 January 2005, and then rescheduled for 12 February 2005, and then moved again (because the White Creek Lodge's lawyers want yet more 'evidence') to 25 May 2005. For the first two of these dates, I'm able to gear myself up to revisit the scene of the crime and defend my moral integrity, with the aid of a close friend who lives in New York City and kindly says she'll be with me every step of the way. I really do feel I need a friend, for one effect of this legal process is to make you vulnerable, easily upset, a toy in their hands. I'm afraid of crumbling, not because this would damage my chance of winning – I've long ago lost interest in anything other than the case being over – but because I don't want the fracture to cause more disintegration in my life than it has already.

The February date is especially awful to contemplate. I fear that Colorado will be full of snow and ice, just as it was four years earlier. We had these conditions briefly in London in the winter of 2003-04, and, when I came out of my office in central London to go home on the first such day, I got to the corner of the street and was reduced to immobility by the little patches of ice on the pavement. I felt sick and started to cry with terror; I had to call a friend to rescue me. I didn't know that the aftermath of a fall could last so long, or take such deep root inside the body.

After the last change of trial date, the White Creek Lodge's attorney offers to settle for $75,000. I say yes; I've never been able to play the game of giving my injury a price tag. The cost to me will never be one that can be wiped out by a dollar cheque. Larry Barnard, predictably, says no. He thinks we can get more. Four months later, they offer a further $25,000. They're resistant, says Larry, to offering even more without seeing me. They want to see if I am actually going to come to the trial. 'You really have to come,' says he: no jury could possibly be expected to be sympathetic to someone who brings a claim without personally attending the trial. I refuse, now, to attend the trial. Now I would have to go alone, since my New York friend must be elsewhere. And I have simply had enough. Larry sends me emails and faxes with YOU MUST ATTEND THE TRIAL in capital letters. Is this harassment, or what? What would have happened if I'd been so badly injured I couldn't travel? I tell him I'll get a medical certificate to prove that attending the trial would be impossible for me. My GP, who seems to be the only one in this who's really on my side, says he'll do (almost) anything to get me out of it. The lawyer manages to annoy him, too, saying he'll come to London to take a deposition from him, and even fixing a day and a time, and then cancelling. It's all a ploy, I later realise, to persuade the White Creek Lodge's lawyer that we are serious. I'm perfectly serious; I want it all to stop. What Larry Barnard is serious about, beyond making money, I really don't know.

My GP is asked for medical reports. The first, written fourteen months post-fracture, notes all the things I still can't do (I give him a list) and records a 'debilitating alteration of sensory perception'. The second medical report, five years post-fracture, just as things hot up with the pre-trial settlement offers, observes that, 'Professor Oakley [my American lawyer never learns to call me this, he persistently uses the incorrect 'Mrs Oakley'] still suffers from a considerable degree of functional impairment...There is little doubt that the extent of the improvement to date is largely a result of Professor Oakley's committed approach to her rehabilitation'. Then they ask him to carry out a more detailed examination, including the 'strength of each motor unit in both upper extremities', bilateral grip strength, and my ability to move my fingers rapidly. He does his best with the equipment available in an ordinary London surgery, and concludes that the impaired functional capacity of my right hand is affected by the persistent sensory loss, and can be measured objectively. But the other side doesn't like this, and they hire a doctor to comment. He calls my GP's report 'a totally inadequate description' and offers to see me to provide a better one, if I fly to the US.

And so it goes on, including the strange story of the scar. They want a photograph of this, and then another one. But I don't care about the scar at all. I can't see it, and even if I could it wouldn't bother me. What bothers me is that I can't feel my right hand. The dissonance here between me and them is that scars are recognised stigmata in American culture, so a dollar tag can be attached to acquiring them. A scar is visible loss of bodily integrity, and damage to bodily integrity is the basis of personal injury claims. Because personal injury claims aren't merely about admission of wrongdoing, but about money, any bodily loss must be measured in pecuniary terms. A hundred years ago, the Miners' Accident Insurance Companies of Germany reckoned that the loss of both hands meant a total inability to earn a living. Separately, the right hand was worth 70%-80% of one's earning capacity: the left hand, 60%-70%. A thumb accounted for 20%-30%. The least useful finger was the third one, only worth 7%-9%.[19] Like amputated fingers, a scar is objectively present: it can be photographed, whereas not being able to feel one's hand is such flimsy evidence, it's hardly evidence at all. The law of evidence in the US is 'probably the most complex, maddening and rule-bound in the entire world'.[20]

Forced into a position in which I have to make it, my own estimate of pecuniary loss is $456,796 for loss of earnings and pension due to having to take early retirement from my job, and not being able to earn money from freelance work for the first few years after the accident. To this I add $11,000 for acupuncture and other therapies; and $7,540 for travel to work because of not being able to ride my bicycle (my usual mode of transport). I should like to add the costs of my time spent attending medical appointments and doing physiotherapy ($218,282), but these are apparently not allowable. There's nothing inflated about these costs; I can show anyone the calculations. My medical costs in the US were paid by my travel insurance, so I only know how much these were when I get copies of my US hospital notes. My four days in hospital ran up a bill of $16,519. The biggest items were the operating room charges ($3,861), 'anesthesia' ($2,621) and medical-surgical supplies ($2,276); the pharmacy notched up an amazing $2,302. I'm so glad I don't live in the USA. I don't enjoy the role of pretending that the real value of life is money.

The American lawyer's main preoccupation in these meaningless computations is, perhaps predictably, with health care costs. I have to explain countless times about the National Health Service. Despite my repeated explanations, Larry Barnard writes to my GP to ask how much my health care has cost. If *I* know the basis of the US health care system, why can't the lawyer who is being paid to take my case know about the NHS? During the telephone deposition, the defence lawyer says he doesn't understand 'the universal health care you have in the UK', and, even after I've explained it yet again, he wants to know whether we pay an extra insurance premium.

The sense of having been allocated a part in someone else's play is strengthened when I get another parcel from the Denver law office. These are legal documents pertaining to something called the 'mounds and obstacles' ruling, a particular speciality of Colorado law designed to protect property owners, such as White Creek Lodge, from too much liability when people fall over and injure themselves on their premises. Larry Barnard wants me to know about this, because it means I should choose my words carefully during the telephone deposition when describing the accident.

The 'mounds and obstacles' ruling dates from a 1957 Colorado High Court decision in the case of *Bonney v Chanter*. On 26 February 1952, Mary Bonney was on her way to work early in the morning when she slipped on the icy pavement in front of a local tax accountant's house. She sued the accountant and won $13,000 in a jury trial, but Justice Clifford of the Colorado High Court later reversed this decision on the basis that landowners have no absolute duty to keep their premises free from ice and snow at all times. Snow and ice are so much part of the climate that such an obligation would be unreasonable. To win such a case, therefore, you have to prove that the snow and ice are more than just superficial: they form mounds which constitute a real obstacle to travel. It's also necessary to establish that the landowner has had enough time to clear the property.

'What exactly did I fall on?', they ask. I remember the ice and the blackness, but I wasn't making an intensive study of the ground at the time. Clare Webb, one of the friends who was with me, took photographs showing lumps of snow intermingled with ice, and I forward these to the lawyer, although whether they're used as evidence, I don't know. 'You MUST NOT mention black ice,' shouts Larry Barnard down the telephone at me. 'DO NOT say the area was generally slippery or snowy.' It isn't hard for me to accept this coaching, because his formulae are entirely consistent with the multiple images in my head. So I write out a form of words which I read when the defence attorney during the deposition asks me to describe the state of the ground: 'The ice was in patches. It was quite lumpy. It looked as though it had been there for some time,' I say. 'Some of the patches were several inches thick.'

Such precision! The defence attorney worries away at it for a while. What was the walkway made of? (How was I supposed to know?) Was there any precipitation that night? (What is 'precipitation'?) Was there any evidence of cinders or salts? I didn't know the answer to this question, either, but I'd been sent a copy of a handwritten statement by Jeff Heller, a White Creek Lodge employee, who recalled the sequence of events as follows: On December 9, the day before the accident, it rained, but in the night the temperature dropped and it snowed. On the morning of December 10, three maintenance men at White Creek Lodge began a 'snow removal and deicing process' which included 'cyndering' [sic] the path on which I fell. During the day the sun came out and melted the snow; then, after the sun went, it started freezing again. When Clare arrived from the airport at 4.30, she pointed out the icy state of the path. Jeff Heller asked one of the maintenance men to go and salt it, but, before he could get there, they had had a call requesting an ambulance to take me to hospital.

Larry Barnard checks the local weather records. There was heavy snow the night of December 9-10, but only flakes during the day. Sunset on December 10 was at 4.36 pm. 'What was the light like that night?' asks the defence lawyer. In my memory, everything is dark and sinister: the sky, the buildings, the ice under my feet. He proceeds, next, to the issue of my culpability: 'Do you remember what you were wearing that night?' We have a confused exchange about trainers ('sneakers') and non-slip (he hears 'non-stick') soles. Was I carrying anything? Had I been on that path before? The defence want to argue that I knew the risk I was taking in walking along that path, so I must also take responsibility for what happened. Another of the defence's questions is about an old back problem which stares out at him from my medical notes. 'It's not a problem, I don't have a problem,' I insist. But he still wants to know what the problem is. I know that what he's getting at here is the moral failure of my body – its ropey skeleton – in causing my arm to break.

Being a litigant is hard, unrewarding work. Only about 15% of the money spent on such cases ever gets through to the injured,[21] and they get less than half of the compensation money awarded.[22] Compensation decisions, whether taken by judges or juries, are based on subjective opinion, which means that exactly the same 'evidence' leads to very different awards being made.[23] We in the UK are no longer safe from some aspects of this pathological legal complexity: a system of conditional fee agreements introduced in 2000 threatens to mimic the inefficiencies of the US system. 'Claim management firms' have taken on the mantle of ambulance-chasers, and are now approaching injury victims directly.[24] This happened in the aftermath of the July 2005 bombings in London. 'Claim handlers' commonly cut deals with insurance companies and lawyers involved in 'no win, no fee' cases charge exhorbitant fees.[25] Where will this 'institutionalized insanity' end? The term comes from Paul Campos's book *Jurismania*, a sustained critique of the US legal system. Campos argues that the system is driven by 'hyperrational modes of decision-making'[26] –

the delusion that the seemingly impersonal objectivity of the legal system can solve all human problems. Lawyers have made this delusion serve their own interests well.

In the end, *Oakley v White Creek Lodge* doesn't go to trial; it's settled out of court, just before the final trial date, like most such cases. Five years and seven months after the accident at White Creek Lodge fractured my arm and my life, I'm sent a cheque with the observation from my US lawyer that, 'It has been a pleasure to be of service to you'.

10

Accidental bodies

The bodies that we're born with, or into, are accidents: unforeseeable chance results of genes, environment, history, time and place. We don't choose our bodies, nor much of what happens to them. But it's difficult to separate the fate of the body and of the self: the two are tied together in the resistance of the body's corporeality, this material package of blood, flesh and bones, wrapped up in a human skin. We have to take our bodies with us on our journey through life, and then, when they don't work any more, we or someone else must decide how to dispose of them: incineration, burial, recycling – the choices are much the same as for any type of rubbish.

Without one of these bodily accidents, the story of *Fracture* would never have happened or been written. My intact right arm couldn't have composed the tale its reconstituted version has: I, the person hiding in the body, would never have had to confront the consequences of skeletal breakdown: the impact on my everyday life, on the relationship between self and body, on the marvellous feats unfractured arms accomplish all the time. Most of all, I wouldn't have been impelled to think about this central paradox of people *having*, but not *being*, bodies. The nature of the connection between body, self, sensation, brain and consciousness would have stayed for me at an abstract level, as theories or opinions more or less arrogantly voiced, more or less believable.

Fracture is my attempt to make sense of what happened to me and my right arm. It's a 'retrospective narratization'[1] which takes the form it does because of my own personal history. The trade of sociological researcher – my trade – implies a certain analytic pose towards both public and private events. What can these tell us about underlying patterns of human social relations, about their successes and failures, about good recipes and bad ones? How can we pass the material of events and situations through a metaphorical sieve, chucking the detritus down the sink, and gazing carefully at the possible gems left behind? There's a certain logic of enquiry in our trade, too: not just *what* happened, but how did different participants *perceive* what happened? What, in people's personal biographies, might account for these perspectives? Are there, perhaps, unanswered questions, puzzles, riddles, wandering about in there that we need to catch hold of and give names to?

There's nothing very unusual about this application of the tools of one's trade to 'biographical disruptions', such as accidents or illness.[2] Connections between the personal and the professional are rife, but often hidden, due to the largely masculine pretence that different areas of one's life should (can) be kept separate. But there are many examples which recognise inseparability, including the 'extended field trip', described earlier in this book, taken by anthropologist Robert Murphy into the culture of his own paralysing illness.[3] *Fracture* is my own field trip: a sociological account of a personal journey into the land of bodily damage, disability and personal injury litigation; a journey taken in a female body with all the additional baggage that implies. Of course, the inseparability of life and work can yield quite different products. For example, David Simpson, a doctor who sustained severe and permanent damage to his right arm and shoulder as a soldier in the Second World War, went on to pioneer the development of powered prosthetic limbs.[4]

For those of us who turn our experience of illness and injury into stories which we offer to others to read, there's the unanswerable question as to how our subjectivity may fashion these narratives in particular ways. If all records of experience are shaped by those who record them (as they are), then we know nothing about the experiences of people whose position in life debars them from participating in such public articulation. Perhaps the body and a sense of self are linked (or not) in many different ways, but we only know about some of these because of the bias in the way knowledge is made.

The more bodies are studied, the more elusive they become.[5] My own search for answers has taken me on different paths. One, quite well-trodden, path, leads though the deceptively bright landscape of modern Western medicine, with its notion of the plastic, programmed body and of people as ill-informed bystanders in a techno-medical system of bodily surveillance and management. Medicine can, and does, save lives and contribute to wellbeing, but much of it is a massive cultural deceit. Its understanding of bodies is limited, and of how people live in bodies even more so. To make up for this lack of comprehension, it promises what it can't deliver: a perfect body, perfectly regulated, existing in perfect harmony with its owner. Our bodies are silent shells, medical mechanisms, or works of art to be sculpted by us in an industry of pushing even further the perfect body project.

A second path trodden by *Fracture* is becoming increasingly popular in social theory and epistemology today, and that's the one which meanders through a maze of interesting questions about bodies and identities. How do bodies shape self-image? What impact, therefore, do changes in the body have on how we think about ourselves? Political discrimination, a major disease on planet earth, is rooted in the body. People are treated differently and unfairly because of the bodies they have. The domination of the globe by white, well-resourced, and so-called 'able-bodied' men means that people of 'other' colours, women and children, the poor, and the 'dis-abled', come off worst. The first basis of social differentiation is what you see. A white male body suggests a certain kind of person. Another kind of person must live in the body of a black pregnant woman. Human prejudice makes bodies determinants of self-image through no fault of their own.

Thirdly, there's this enduring, frightening, question of how we know our bodies in the world. Without the body, we can know only about our own consciousness. But the body's positional knowledge of itself can only be communicated through 'cutaneous sensibility', and this, despite the efforts of modern neurophysiology, remains a pretty mysterious thing.[6] How do receptors in the skin respond to external stimuli and interact to yield those intricate and complex perceptions which indicate when (in one of the many senses in which we use that word) we say we 'feel' something? The body is how we know the world, but its interaction with the environment through the skin is meaningless to us unless messages both pass from the skin to our brain and are correctly decoded by us. In a postmodern world, the idea of 'correct decoding' may be seen as redundant, yet in practice many aspects of life would be impossible without this smooth alliance between body and self in producing positional knowledge. Paralysed bodies are the most extreme example. The relatively trivial accident of a partially paralysed hand merely offers a clue as to what this kind of loss 'feels' – or more accurately doesn't 'feel' – like.

You only know it works when it doesn't work any more. This is how I was precipitated into my personal journey down these paths, and how I came to ask the questions this book tangles with about the puzzle of human embodiment. The fracture which followed the White Creek Lodge's lack of attention to its icy paths left me with a disability neither I nor the doctors who treated me understood. We still don't know the causes of the failure of part of my right hand to feel. Even putting it like that asserts an answer that may be false. Is the failure really one of the hand itself, or is it of the brain's capacity to notice what the hand is feeling? And, as the person stitching all these organs together, what responsibility do I have for what it seems none of us can cure? The last of these questions has a particular resonance in a culture which ascribes moral responsibility to each one of us for her or his own health.[7] The breakdown of the perfect body project is at least partly a question of our own personal negligence, a viewpoint which was at the forefront of the defence lawyers' minds in my own legal case against White Creek Lodge. Moral chaos and incapacity join physical suffering and dis-ability as consequences of bodily accidents.

There are two main ways in which the experience of

bodily disorder is described in Western culture: as 'pain' and as 'suffering'. Yet these are clumsy, inadequate and misleading terms for explaining how it feels to live in a disordered body. 'Suffering' appeals to the image of dependent patients and sends them as supplicants to the superior ministry of medicine. 'Pain' is bodily suffering, the punishment meted out to the person within. But you can experience accidents and illness without being jettisoned into a state of dependent patienthood, and many sensations which accompany illness and injury are different and disturbing without being, simply, painful.

Many times during the writing of this book, I've reflected on the observation that 'nerves' are a dominant form of suffering and cause of patienthood in Western culture.[8] This is especially the case for women, whose close association with their bodies has made their identities and self-images much more contingent on bodily state than is the case for men. Women's bodies have traditionally been seen as reducing them to states of nervous frenzy, hysteria or lassitude – as, indeed, driving them mad. Perhaps there's no more complete condition of bodily alienation than femininity. The cultural illness of being a woman invades the body and the self; there's just no escape from it. On the other hand, there are lots of pills, medicaments and ways of medical seeing that can help. Science returns us, not to our genes, but to the illusions of gender and science themselves.

Writing is a way to assert the authenticity of the self. This is undoubtedly one explanation as to why *Fracture* came to be written. The assertion of writing is doubly necessary for a writer and for someone whose dominant right hand has been hurt. Through text, we reclaim the body; we have some hope of owning and integrating the experience of damage. This is necessarily a self-absorbed act. It makes us focus on the self, because it's the self that we feel has been assaulted, and will remain under attack unless, like Humpty Dumpty, we pick up the broken pieces and put them together again. An unfortunate consequence of this unattractively solipsistic task is that other people's viewpoints get eclipsed. The story of *Fracture* as told here has excised the critically important roles other people played in the aftermath of my injury, and it hasn't even begun to acknowledge how *they* may have felt about these uninvited calls on their time and attention, which were met with love and generosity. This is true of my family and friends, and my work colleagues. It's also startingly true of the two friends who were with me when the accident happened, and without whose selfless care – their forced precipitation out of a much needed holiday into a 'vast, medicalised space' – I would never have been in a position to write this book. It's not a justification, but an explanation, to say that writing a story which is democratically faithful to the perspectives of everyone in it is a different enterprise from the self-centred act of writing to unite the elements of a fractured self.

Fracture has taken me four years to write, years in which writing – mostly by hand – has been both a challenge and a constant reminder of the event commemorated in its title. Using a pencil, which the British Library now insists on, to take notes from books, nearly defeated me at one point, and certainly seemed literally to add insult to injury. Still today the act of writing, with any kind of implement, or on the computer, can't be undertaken without my consciousness of the deficient sensation of my right hand. When I write by hand, I know my hand rests on the paper and moves across it as the ink or the lead inscribe words, because I can see it and them there, but its own perception of the surface beneath it is dim, at best. The paper could be concrete or velvet, silk or gravel; only my eyes can tell. After a while writing, all sensation in that part of my hand disappears, and two of my fingers, part of the back of my hand and the skin journeying across the paper become totally insensitive and cold. When I use the computer, the affected part of my hand becomes first cold, then, after about ten minutes, it retreats into numbness, and the clawing of the last two fingers starts to return. Thanks to my wonderful physiotherapist, I can still hold the pen, or tap the keyboard and operate the mouse through this numbness and insensitivity. But the legend of the textbooks has come, and remains, true: I have function, but not sensation. I can only say that any experience of the world devoid of sensation isn't much worth having.

In his journey through opium addiction, Jean Cocteau remarked, 'Superficiality is the only crime. Everything that is understood is right'.[9] If there's too much complexity, too much probing beneath the surface of things in this book, I apologise. For me, it was necessary to the goal of understanding. I would like to think that my journey towards this goal has uncovered commonalities in the human experience of embodiment and problems of health, illness and the body in our culture we need to address, and even some tentative ways forward in the physiology and neurology of identity.

Notes

Chapter 1

1   Ackland, D. and Freeburg, J. (1988) *The Rockies*, Singapore: APA Publications.

Chapter 2

1   The title is borrowed from the landmark volume *Our bodies, ourselves* (1973), prepared by the Boston Women's Health Book Collective, New York: Simon and Schuster.
2   Manderson, L. (2002) 'My left arm: experiencing brachial plexoplathy', *Internal Medicine Journal*, vol 32, no 7, pp 353-356.
3   Ralston, A. (2004) *Between a rock and a hard place*, London: Pocket Books, pp 25-26, pp 279, 299.
4   Turner, B.S. (1984) *The body and society*, Oxford: Basil Blackwell, p 7.
5   Leder, D. (1992) 'The Cartesian corpse and the lived body', in D. Leder (ed.) *The body in medical thought and practice*, Dordrecht: Kluwer Academic, p 25.
6   Leder, D. (1990) *The absent body*, Chicago: University of Chicago Press.
7   d'Houtaud, A. and Field, M.G. (1984) 'The image of health: variations in perception by social class in a French population', *Sociology of Health and Illness*, vol 6, no 1, pp 30-60.
8   Grosz, E. (1992) 'Bodies-cities', in B. Columbia (ed.) *Sexuality and space*, New York: Princeton Architectural Press, p 243.

9   Grealy, L. (2004) *Autobiography of a face*, London: Methuen.

10 Williams, S.J. and Bendelow, G. (1998) *The lived body: Sociological themes, embodied issues,* London: Routledge, p 160.

11 Draaisma, D. (2004) *Why life speeds up as you get older: How memory shapes our past,* Cambridge: Cambridge University Press,

12 Brison, S.J. (2002) *Aftermath: Violence and the remaking of a self,* Princeton, N.J.: Princeton University Press.

13 Raine, N.V. (1999) *After silence: Rape and my journey back,* London: Virago.

14 Wynn Parry, C.B. (1981) *Rehabilitation of the hand* (4th edn), London: Butterworths, p 90.

15 Brand, P.W. (1987) 'The hand in leprosy', in D.W. Lamb (ed.) *The paralysed hand,* Edinburgh: Churchill Livingstone.

16 King, S. (2000) *On writing,* London: Hodder and Stoughton, p 219.

17 Botton, G. (1999) *The therapeutic potential of creative writing,* London: Jessica Kingsley, p 20.

18 Manning, R. (1987) *A corridor of mirrors,* London: The Women's Press, p 165.

19 Botton, p 199.

20 Brison.

21 Cocteau, J. (1933) (trans. E. Boyd) *The diary of an addict,* London: Allen and Unwin, p 12.

22 Greenhalgh, T. (1999) 'Narrative-based medicine in an evidence-based world', *British Medical Journal,* vol 318, pp 323-325.

23 Cocteau, p 177.

24 Fairhurst, E. (1977) 'On being a patient in an orthopaedic ward: some thoughts on the definition of the situation', in A. Davis and G. Horobin (eds) *Medical encounters,* London: Croom Helm, p 160.

25 Steedman, C. (2000) 'Enforced narrative: stories of another self', in T. Cosslett, C. Lury and P. Summerfield (eds) *Feminism and autobiography,* London: Routledge, p 25.

26 Grosz, E. (1994) *Volatile bodies: Toward a corporeal feminism,* Bloomington: Indiana University Press.

27 Oakley, A. (1980) *Women confined: Towards a sociology of childbirth,* Oxford: Martin Robertson.

28 Marris, P. (1996, revised edition) *Loss and change,* London: Routledge, p 147.

29 Becker, G. (1997) *Disrupted lives: How people create meaning in a chaotic world,* Berkeley: University of California Press.

30 Fisher, S.H. (1960) 'Psychiatric considerations of hand disability', *Archives of Physical Medicine and Rehabilitation,* vol 41, pp 62-70, pp 68-69.

31 Giddens, A. (1991) *The consequences of modernity,* Cambridge: Polity Press.

32 Brison, p 16.

33 Lovell, A., Zander, L.I., James, C.E., Foot, S., Swan, A.V. and Reynolds, A. (1987) 'The St Thomas's Hospital maternity case-notes study: a randomised controlled trial to assess the effects of giving expectant mothers their own maternity case-notes', *Paediatric and Perinatal Epidemiology,* vol 1, pp 55-66.

34 Heilbrun, C. (1989) *Writing a woman's life,* London: The Women's Press.

35 http://archives.cnn.com/2000/HEALTH/10/20/hand.transplant.ap/index.html, accessed 16 April 2006.

Chapter 3

1 Sacks, O. (1990) *A leg to stand on,* London: HarperCollins, p 186, p 98.

2 Sacks, p 52.

3 Leder, D. (1990) *The absent body,* Chicago: University of Chicago Press, p 149.

4 Murray, E., Burns, J., Tai See, E., Lai, R. and Nazareth, I. (2005) 'Interactive Health Communication Applications for people with chronic disease', *The Cochrane Database of Systematic Reviews,* Issue 4, Art.No:CD004274.DOI:10.1002/1465858.CDOO4274.pub4.

5 Wynn Parry, C.B. (1981) *Rehabilitation of the hand* (4th edn), London: Butterworths, p 78.

6 Sacks, O. (1985) *The man who mistook his wife for a hat,* London: Gerald Duckworth, p 1.

7 Galbraith, K.A., McCullough, C.J. (1979) 'Acute nerve injury as a complication of closed fractures or dislocations of the elbow', *Injury,* vol 11, no 2, pp 1599-1664.

8 Head, H. in conjunction with Rivers, W.H.R., Sherren, J., Holmes, G., Thompson, I. and Riddoch, G. (1920) *Studies in neurology* (2 vols.), London: Henry Frowde, and Hodder and Stoughton.

9 Henson, R.A. (1961) 'Henry Head's work on sensation', in K.W. Gross, R.A. Henson, M. Critchley and R. Brain (eds) *Henry Head: Essays and bibliography,* London: Macmillan.

10 Slobodin, R. (1987) *Rivers,* Stroud, Glos.: Sutton Publishing Ltd, p 32.

11 Head, p 125.

12 Head, p 192.

13 Kevles, D.J. (1985) *In the name of eugenics,* New York: Alfred A Knopf.

14 Head, p 276.

15 Boscheinen-Morrin, J., Davey, V. and Conolly, W.B. (1985) *The hand: Fundamentals of therapy,* London: Butterworths.

16 Wynn Parry, p 84.

17 Callaghan, A.D. (1987) 'Role of the therapist in rehabilitation of the paralysed hand', in D.W. Lamb (ed.) *The paralysed hand,* Edinburgh: Churchill Livingstone, p 245

18 Skrover, T. (1992) 'Nerve injuries', in B.G. Stanley and S.M. Tribuzi (eds) *Concepts in hand rehabilitation,* Philadelphia: F.A. Davis, p 324.

19 Head, pp 99-100, p 30.

20 Ruijs, A.C., Jaquet, J.B., Kalmijn, S., Gielc, H. and Hovins, S.R. (2005) 'Median and ulnar nerve injuries: a meta-analysis of predictors of motor and sensory recovery after modern microsurgical nerve repair', *Plastic and Reconstructive Surgery,* vol 116, no 2, pp 484-494.

21 Henson.

22 Leont'ev, A.N. and Zaporozhets, A.V. (1960, originally published 1945) *Rehabilitation of hand function* (trans. B. Haigh, W. Ritchie Russell (ed.)), Oxford: Oxford University Press, p 14.

23 Brown, P.H. (1987) 'Introduction', in D.W. Lamb (ed.) *The paralysed hand,* Edinburgh: Churchill Livingstone, p 5.

24 Leont'ev and Zaporozhets, p 47.

25 Leont'ev and Zaporozhets, p 46.

26 Miller, J. (2000, originally published 1978) *The body in question,* London: Pimlico, p 7.

27 Enna, C.D. (1988) *Peripheral denervation of the hand.* New York: Alan R Liss Inc., p 35.
28 Miller.
29 Rosen, B., Lundborg, G., Dahlin, L.B., Holmberg, J. and Karlson, B. (1994) 'Nerve repair: correlation of restitution of functional sensibility with specific cognitive capacities', *Journal of Hand Surgery,* vol 19, no 4, pp 454-458, p 455.
30 Sacks, 1985, p x.
31 Ruijs et al., p 484.
32 Sacks, 1985, p 46.
33 Rosen et al., p 455.
34 Björkman, A., Rosen, B. and Lundborg, G. (2004) 'Acute improvement of hand sensibility after selective ipsilateral cutaneous forearm anaesthesia', *European Journal of Neuroscience,* vol 20, pp 2733-2736, p 2735.
35 Dellon, A.L. (1981) *Evaluation of sensibility and re-education of sensation in the hand,* Baltimore: Williams and Wilkins, p 98.
36 Meuse, S. (1996) 'Phantoms, lost limbs, and the limits of the body-self', in M. O'Donovan-Anderson (ed.) *The incorporated self: Interdisciplinary perspectives on embodiment,* Lanham, Maryland: Rowman and Littlefield Publishers.

Chapter 4

1 Burdick, L.D. (1905) *The hand: A survey of facts, legends and beliefs pertaining to manual ceremonies, covenants and symbols,* New York: The Irving Company.

2   van den Berg, J.H. (1952) 'The human body and the significance of human movement', *Philosophy and Phenomenological Research*, vol 13, p 169 (cited in D. Leder (1990) *The absent body*, Chicago: University of Chicago Press, p 1).

3   Bowers, W.H. and Tribuzi, S.M. (1992) 'Functional anatomy', in B.G. Stanley and S.M. Tribuzi (eds) *Concepts in hand rehabilitation*, Philadelphia: F.A. Davis, pp 3, 33.

4   Bell, C. (1874, originally published 1832) *The hand: Its mechanism and vital endowments, as evincing design* (9th edn), London: George Bell and Sons, p 15.

5   Tabori, P. (1962) *The book of the hand: A compendium of fact and legend since the dawn of history*, Philadelphia and New York: Chilton Co., p 16.

6   Berry, T.J. (1963) *The hand as a mirror of systemic disease*, Philadelphia: FA Davis Company, p x.

7   Fisher, S.H. (1960) 'Psychiatric considerations of hand disability', *Archives of Physical Medicine and Rehabilitation*, vol 41, pp 62-70, p 64.

8   Brown, E. (2002) 'The prosthetics of management: Motion study, photography and the industrialized body in World War I America', in K. Ott, D. Serlin and S. Mihm (eds) *Artificial parts, practical lives*, New York: New York University Press.

9   Lister, G. (1993) *The hand: Diagnosis and indications* (3rd edn), Edinburgh: Churchill Livingstone, p 1.

10 Berry, p x.

11 Solzhenitsyn, A. (1979) *The first circle* (trans. M. Guybon), London: Fontana, p 640.

12 Barr, N.R. and Swan, D. (1988) *The hand: Principles and techniques of splint making*, London: Butterworths, p 18.

13 Burdick, p 142.

14 Springer, S.P. and Deutsch, G. (1993) *Left brain, right brain*, New York: W.H. Freeman, p 128.

15 Barr and Swan, p 1.

16 Hertz, R. (1960, originally published 1907 and 1909) *Death and the right hand* (trans. R. Needham and C. Needham), Aberdeen: Cohen and West, p 89.

17 Chelhod, J. (1973) 'A contribution to the problem of the pre-eminence of the right, based upon Arabian evidence', in R. Needham (ed.) *Right and left: Essays on dual symbolic classification*, Chicago: University of Chicago Press, p 239.

18 Evans-Pritchard, E.E. (1973) 'Nuer spear symbolism', in R. Needham (ed.) *Right and left: Essays on dual symbolic classification*, Chicago: University of Chicago Press.

19 'Left hand, right hand' (editorial) (1981) *British Medical Journal*, vol 282, p 588.

20 Beidelman, T.O. (1973) 'Kaguru symbolic classification', in R. Needham (ed.) *Right and left: Essays on dual symbolic classification*, Chicago: University of Chicago Press.

21 Evans-Pritchard.

22 Sagan, C. (1978) *The dragons of Eden*, London: Hodder and Stoughton.

23 Beidelman, p 135.

24 Burdick, p 148.

25 Granet, M. (1973) 'Right and left in China', in R. Needham (ed.) *Right and left: Essays on dual symbolic classification*, Chicago: University of Chicago Press.

26 Lindenbaum, S. (1968) 'Women and the left hand: social status and symbolism in East Pakistan', *Mankind*, vol 6, no 11, pp 537-544.

27 Tabori, p 184.

28 http://en.wikopedia.org/wiki/Rick_Allen (Def_Leppard_drummer), accessed 26 August 2006.

29 Hertz, p 103.

30 http://onin.com/fp/fphistory.html, accessed 11 June 2006.

31 http://en.wikipedia.org/wiki/Fingerprint, accessed 11 June 2006.

32 Warren-Davis, O. (1993) *The hand reveals*, Longmead, Shaftesbury, Dorset: Element Books.

33 McManus, C. (2002) *Right hand, left hand: The origins of asymmetry in brains, bodies, atoms and cultures*, London: Weidenfeld and Nicholson, p 156.

34 McManus, p 125.

35 Beidelman, pp 151-152.

36 Hertz, p 98.

37 McManus, p 154.

38 Springer, pp 1-2.

39 McManus, p. 191.

40 McManus, p 144.

41 McManus, p 234.

42 Ramadhani, M.K., Elias, S.G., van Noord, P.A.H., Grobbee, D.E., Peeters, P.H.M. and Uiterwaal, C.S.P.M. (2005) 'Innate left-handedness and risk of breast cancer: case-cohort study', *British Medical Journal*, vol 331, pp 882-883.

43 Berry, p 150.

44 Wynn Parry, C.B. (1981) *Rehabilitation of the hand* (4th ed), London: Butterworths, p 1.

45 Parry, p 78.

46 Parry, p 91.

47 McManus, p 35.

48 Cited in McManus, p 257.

Chapter 5

1 Woolf, V. (1967, originally published in 1930) 'On being ill', in *Collected essays* (vol 4), London: The Hogarth Press, pp 193-4.

2 Kleinman, A. (1988) *The illness narratives*, New York: Basic Books. See also Aronson, J.K. (2000) 'Authopathography: the patient's tale', *British Medical Journal*, vol 321, pp 1599-1602.

3 Toombs, S.K. (1992) 'The body in multiple sclerosis: a patient's perspective', in D. Leder (ed) *The body in medical thought and practice*, Dordrecht/ Boston/London: Kluwer Academic, p 127.

4 Pillsbury, G. (2001) 'Refusing to fight: a playful approach to chronic disease', in S. Cunningham-Burley and K. Backett-Milburn (eds) *Exploring the body*, Houndsmill, Basingstoke, Hampshire: Palgrave, p 70.

5 Cocteau, J. (1933) (trans. E. Boyd) *Opium: The diary of an addict*, London: Allen and Unwin, p 97.

6 Toombs, p 127.

7 Mairs, N. (1997) 'Carnal acts', in K. Conboy, N. Medina and S. Stanbury (eds) *Writing on the body: Female embodiment and feminist theory*, New York: Columbia University Press, p 298.

8 Pillsbury, p 65.

9 Williams, S.J. (1996) 'The vicissitudes of embodiment across the chronic illness trajectory', *Body and Society*, vol 21, no 2, pp 23-24.

10 Seymour, W. (1989) *Bodily alterations*, Sydney: Allen and Unwin, p 80.

11 Macintyre, S. and Oldman, D. (1977) 'Coping with migraine', in A. Davis and G. Horobin (eds) *Medical encounters*, London: Croom Helm.

12 Richardson, J.C. (2005) 'Establishing the (extra)ordinary in chronic widespread pain', *Health: An Interdisciplinary Journal for the Social Study of Health, Illness and Medicine,* vol 9, no 1, pp 31-48.

13 Lowton, L. and Gabe, J. (2003) 'Life on a slippery slope: perceptions of health in adults with cystic fibrosis', *Sociology of Health and Illness,* vol 25, no 4, pp 289-319.

14 Brinson, P. and Dick, F. (1996) *Fit to dance? The Report of the National Inquiry into Dancers' Health and Injury,* London: Calouste Gulbenkian Foundation.

15 Turner, B.S. and Wainwright, S.P. (2003) 'Corps de ballet: the case of the injured ballet dancer', *Sociology of Health and Illness,* vol 25, no 4, pp 269-288.

16 Strong, P. (1977) 'Medical errands: a discussion of routine patient work', in A. Davis and G. Horobin (eds) *Medical encounters,* London: Croom Helm, p 42.

17 McGrath, M. (2002) *Silvertown: An East End family memoir,* London: Fourth Estate, pp 62-67.

18 Seymour, p 11.

19 Burnett, K.A. and Holmes, M. (2001) 'Bodies, battlefields and biographies: scars and the construction of the body as heritage', in S. Cunningham-Burley and K. Backett-Milburn (eds) *Exploring the body,* Houndsmill, Basingstoke, Hampshire: Palgrave.

20 van der Ker, A.L., Conori, L.U.M., Smeulders, M.J.C., Draajers, L.J., van der Horst, C.M.A.M. and van Zmijlen, P.D.M. (2005) 'Reliable and feasible evaluation of linear scars by the Patient and Observer Scar Assessment Scale', *Plastic and Reconstructive Surgery,* vol 116, no 2, pp 514-522.

21 Taylor, L. (1982) 'Preface', in M. Hepworth and M. Featherstone *Surviving middle age,* Oxford: Basil Blackwell.

22 Illich, I. (1992) *In the mirror of the past: Lectures and addresses 1978-90,* New York and London: Marion Boyars.

23 Kalodner, C.R. (2003) *Too fat or too thin? A reference guide to eating disorders,* Westport, Conn: Greenwood Press, p 51.

24 Cash, T.F. and Deagle, E.A. (1997) 'The nature and extent of body-image disturbances in anorexia nervosa and bulimia nervosa: a meta-analysis', *International Journal of Eating Disorders,* vol 22, no 2, pp 107-126.

25 Kalodner, p 10, p 3.

26 Furman, F.K. (1997) *Facing the mirror: Older women and beauty shop culture,* London: Routledge.

27 Miller, J.B. (1976) *Toward a new psychology of women,* Boston: Beacon Press.

28 Howson, A. (2005) *Embodying gender,* London: Sage.

29 Chapkis, W. (1986) *Beauty secrets: Women and the politics of appearance,* London: The Women's Press.

30 Murphy, Y. and Murphy, R.F. (1974) *Women of the forest,* New York: Columbia University Press.

31 Murphy, R.F. (1987) *The body silent,* London: J.M. Dent, p ix.

32 Goffman, E. (1990) *Stigma: Notes on the management of spoiled identity,* London: Penguin.

33 Good, B.J. (1994) *Medicine, rationality and experience,* Cambridge: Cambridge University Press, p 117.

34 Sarton, M. (1988) *After the stroke,* London: The Women's Press, p 75.

35 Murphy, p 75.

Chapter 6

1 Porter, R. (2002) *Blood and guts: A short history of medicine*, London: Allen Lane, p 55.
2 Sawday, J. (1995) *The body emblazoned: Dissection and the human body in Renaissance culture*, London: Routledge, p 10.
3 Leder, D. (1990) *The absent body*, Chicago: University of Chicago Press, p 146.
4 Armstrong, D. (1983) *Political anatomy of the body*, Cambridge: Cambridge University Press.
5 Good, B.J. (1994) *Medicine, rationality and experience*, Cambridge: Cambridge University Press, p 8.
6 Young, K. (1997) *Presence in the flesh: The body in medicine*, Harvard: Harvard University Press.
7 Arney, W.R. and Bergen, B.J. (1983) 'The anomaly, the chronic patient and the play of medical power', *Sociology of Health and Illness*, vol 5, no 1, pp 1-24.
8 Rosenfield, I. (1992) *The strange, familiar and forgotten*, London: Picador, p 14.
9 Sawday.
10 Toombs, S.K. (1992) 'The body in multiple sclerosis: a patient's perspective', in D. Leder (ed.) *The body in medical thought and practice*, Dordrecht/Boston/London: Kluwer Academic, p 133.
11 Sacks, O. (1990) *A leg to stand on*, London: HarperCollins.
12 Scarry, E. (1985) *The body in pain: The making and unmaking of the world*, New York: Oxford University Press, p 4.
13 Arney and Bergen.
14 Wall, P. (1999) *Pain: The science of suffering*, London: Weidenfeld and Nicolson.

15 Williams, S.J. and Bendelow, G. (1998) *The lived body: Sociological themes, embodied issues,* London: Routledge.

16 Miller, J. (2000, originally published in 1978) *The body in question,* London: Random House, p 14.

17 Pillsbury, G. (2001) 'Refusing to fight: a playful approach to chronic disease', in S. Cunningham-Burley and K. Backett-Milburn (eds) *Exploring the body,* Houndsmill, Basingstoke, Hampshire: Palgrave, p 62.

18 Kinzman, S. (2002) '"There's no language for this". Communication and alignment in contemorary prosthetics', in K. Ott, D. Serlin and S. Milim (eds) *Artificial parts, practical lives,* New York: New York University Press.

19 Tinel, J. (2005) '"Tingling" signs with peripheral nerve injury', *La Prise Médicale,* vol 47 (1915) pp 388-389, trans. *The Journal of Hand Surgery,* vol 30B, no 1, pp 87-89, p 87.

20 Wynn Parry, C.B. (1981) *Rehabilitation of the hand* (4th edn), London: Butterworths, p 128.

21 Stanley, B.G. and Tribuzi, S.M. (1992) *Concepts in hand rehabilitation,* Philadelphia: F.A. Davis, p 107.

22 Ruijs, A.C., Jaquet, J.B., Kalmijn, S., Giele, H and Hovius, S.R. (2005) 'Median and ulnar nerve injuries: a meta-analysis of predictors of motor and sensory recovery after modern microsurgical repair', *Plastic and Reconstructive Surgery,* vol 116, no 2, pp 484-494.

23 Brown, P.W. (1987) 'Introduction', in D. Lamb (ed.) *The paralyzed hand,* Edinburgh: Churchill Livingstone, p 8.

24 Sacks, O. (1985) *The man who mistook his wife for a hat,* London: Gerald Duckworth, p 46.

25 Moran, C.A. and Callahan, A.D. (1986) 'Sensibility measurement and management', in C.A. Moran (ed.) *Hand rehabilitation*, New York: Churchill Livingstone, pp 45-46.

26 Moran and Callahan, p 58.

27 Rosen, B., Lundborg, G., Dahlin, L.B., Holmberg, J. and Karlsson, B. (1994) 'Nerve repair: correlation of restitution of functional sensibility with specific cognitive capacities', *Journal of Hand Surgery*, vol 19, no 4, pp 452-458, p 455.

28 Merzenrich, M.M., Jenkins, W.M. and Keck, U.M. (1993) 'Reorganization of cortical representations of the hand following alterations of skin inputs induced by nerve injury, skin island transfers and experiences', *Journal of Hand Therapy*, vol 6, no 2, pp 89-104, p 89.

29 Moran and Callahan.

30 Rosen et al., p 452.

31 Sacks, O. (1995) *An anthropologist on Mars*, London: Picador, p 132.

32 Vega-Bermundez, F. and Johnson, K.O. (2002) 'Spatial acuity after digit amputation', *Brain*, vol 125, no 6, pp 1256-1264.

33 Seymour, W. (1989) *Bodily alterations*, Sydney: Allen and Unwin.

34 Dellon, p 221.

35 Moran and Callahan, p 46.

36 Bendelow, G.A. and Williams, S.J. (1995) 'Transcending the dualisms: towards a sociology of pain', *Sociology of Health and Illness*, vol 17, no 2, pp 139-165.

37 Head, p 243.

38 Vickers, A. (2001) 'Acupuncture', *Effective Health Care Bulletin*, vol 7, no 2, University of York: NHS Centre for Reviews and Dissemination.

39 http://www.ultdentist.com/gemtherapy.htm, accessed 16 June 2003; http://en.mimi.hu/jewelry/carnelian.html, accessed 11 July 2006.

40 http://www.senderogroup.com/mikejournal.htm, 23 April 2000, accessed 17 April 2006.

41 Abrams, M. (2002) 'Sight unseen', *The Braille Monitor*, November. http://www.nfb.org/bm/bm02/bm0211/bm021105.htm, accessed 17 April 2006.

42 Abrams, p 6.

43 Vickers.

44 Becker, G. (1997) *Disrupted lives: How people create meaning in a chaotic world*, Berkeley: University of California Press, p 39.

45 Woolf, V. (1967, originally published in 1930) 'On being ill', in *Collected essays* (vol 4), London: The Hogarth Press.

46 Dellon, p ix.

47 Braune, S. and Schady, W. (1993) 'Changes in sensation after nerve injury or amputation: the role of central factors', *Journal of Neurology, Neurosurgery and Psychiatry*, vol 56, pp 393-399, p 393.

48 Cocteau, pp 12-13.

49 McCabe, C.S., Haigh, R.C., Ring, E.F.J., Halligan, P.W., Wall, P.D. and Blake, D.R. (2003) 'A controlled pilot study of the utility of mirror visual feedback in the treatment of complex regional pain syndrome', *Rheumatology* vol 42, pp 97-101.

50 Shenker, N.G.N. and Blake, D.R. (2002) 'Understanding pain: the enigma of pain and suffering', *Royal College of Physicians' Journal*, vol 2, Nov/Dec.

51 Dean, L. (2005) 'Rehabilitation of an ulnar nerve lesion following elbow fracture: A single case study', Integrated Musculoskeletal Trauma Conference, Belfast, Ireland.

Chapter 7

1   Schiebinger, L. (1993) *Nature's body*, London: HarperCollins.

2   Klinge, I. (1998) *Gender and bones: The production of osteoporosis 1941-96*, Utrecht: University of Utrecht.

3   Albright, F., Smith, P.H. and Richardson, A.M. (1941) 'Postmenopausal osteoporosis: its clinical features', *Journal of the American Medical Association*, vol 116, pp 2465-2474.

4   Drife, J.O. (1992) 'Are breasts redundant organs?' in R. Holland (ed.) *Soundings from BMJ columnists*, London: BMJ Publishing Group.

5   Clark, J. (2003) 'A hot flush for Big Pharma', *British Medical Journal*, vol 327, p 400.

6   Clark.

7   Burgermeister, J. (2003) 'Head of German medicines body likens HRT to thalidomide', *British Medical Journal*, vol 327, p 767.

8   Moynihan, R., Bero, L., Ross-Degnan, D., Henry, D., Lee, K., Watkins, J., Mah, C. and Soumerai, S.B. (2000) 'Coverage by the news media of the benefits and risks of medications', *New England Journal of Medicine*, vol 342, pp 1645-1650.

9   Clark.

10 Jolleys, J.V. and Olesen, F. (1996) 'A comparative study of prescribing hormone replacement therapy in the USA and Europe', *Maturitas*, vol 23, no 1, pp 47-53.

11 Hemminki, E. and Topo, P. (1997) 'Prescribing of hormone therapy in menopause and postmenopause', *Journal of Psychosomatic Obstetrics and Gynecology*, vol 18, pp 145-157.

12 Sand, G. cited in G. Sheehy (1992) *The silent passage,* New York: Random House, p 32.

13 Barrett-Connor, E. (1998) 'Hormone replacement therapy', *British Medical Journal,* vol 317, pp 457-461, p 457.

14 Martin, E. (1987) *The woman in the body,* Boston: Beacon Press, p 173.

15 Klinge, p 73.

16 Klinge, p 50.

17 Klinge, pp 70-71.

18 Cadogan, J., Eastell, R., Jones, M. and Barker, M.E. (1997) 'Milk intake and bone mineral acquisition in adolescent girls: randomised, controlled intervention trial', *British Medical Journal,* vol 315, pp 1255-1260, p 1255.

19 Francis, R.M. (2000) 'The increasing use of peripheral bone densitometry', (editorial) *British Medical Journal,* vol 321, pp 396-398.

20 Charatan, F. (2002) 'The great American mammography debate', *British Medical Journal,* vol 324, p 432.

21 Roberts, M. (1989) 'Breast screening: time for a rethink', *British Medical Journal,* vol 299, pp 1153-55; Baines, C.J. (2005) 'Rethinking breast screening again', *British Medical Journal,* vol 331, p 1031.

22 Raffle, A.R., Alden, B., Quinn, M., Babb, P.J. and Brett, M.T. (2003) 'Outcome of screening to prevent cancer: analysis of cumulative incidence of cervical abnormality and modelling of cases and deaths prevented', *British Medical Journal,* vol 326, pp 901-904.

23 Thornton, H. and Dixon-Woods, M. (2002) 'Prostate specific antigen testing for prostate cancer', *British Medical Journal,* vol 325, pp 725-726.

24 Fenton, J.J. and Elmore, J.G. (2004) 'Balancing mammography's benefits and risks', *British Medical Journal*, vol 328: E301-E302.

25 Jørgensen, K.J.. and Gøtzsche, P.C. (2006) 'Content of invitations for publicly funded screening mammography', *British Medical Journal*, vol 332, pp 538-541.

26 Yamey, G. and Wilkes, M. (2002) 'The PSA storm', *British Medical Journal*, vol 324, p 431.

27 Lu-Yao, G., Albertsen, P.C., Stanford, J.L., Stukel, T.A., Corkery, E.S. and Barry, M.J. (2002) 'Natural experiment examining impact of aggressive screening and treatment on prostate cancer mortality in two fixed cohorts from Seattle area and Connecticut', *British Medical Journal*, vol 325, pp 740-745.

28 Tuck, S.P. and Francis, R.M. (2002) 'Osteoporosis', *Postgraduate Medical Journal*, vol 78, pp 526-532, p 526.

29 Pearce, K.E. (2000) 'Osteoporosis is a risk factor, not a disease', *British Medical Journal*, vol 322, p 862.

30 Derman, R. (2003) 'Identifying the osteopenic patient and preventing worsening of the disease', *Current Women's Health Reports*, vol 3, pp 199-206.

31 Mitchell, D., Johnell, O. and Welch, H. (1996) 'Meta-analysis of how well measures of BMD predict occurrence of osteoporotic fractures', *British Medical Journal*, vol 312, pp 1254-1259.

32 Mayor, S. (2002) 'Review warns that risks of long-term HRT outweigh benefits', *British Medical Journal*, vol 325, p 673.

33 McPherson, K. (2004) 'Where are we now with hormone replacement therapy?' *British Medical Journal*, vol 328, pp 357-358.

34 *Sensible News*, May 2005.

35 Black, D., Schwartz, A., Enstrud, K., Rybak-Feiglin, A., Gupta, J., Lombardi, A., Wallace, R., Levis, S., Quandt, S., Satterfield, S., Cauley, J. and Cummings, S. (2004) '5 year randomized trial of the long-term efficacy and safety of alendronate', *Journal of Bone Mineral Research*, vol 10 (Suppl 1): S45.

36 Ott, S.M. (2005) 'Long-term safety of bisphosphonates', *The Journal of Clinical Endocrinology and Metabolism*, vol 90, no 3, pp 1897-1899.

37 Kannus, P., Dalvanen, M., Kaprio, J., Parkkan, J. and Koskenvo, M. (1999) 'Genetic factors and osteoporotic fractures in elderly people: prospective 25 year follow up of a nationwide cohort of elderly Finnish twins', *British Medical Journal*, vol 319, pp 1334-1337.

38 Wilkin, T.J. (2001) 'Bone densitometry is not a good predictor of hip fracture', *British Medical Journal*, vol 323, pp 795-799.

39 Coupland, C.A.C., Cliffe, S.J., Bassey, E.J., Grainge, M.J., Hosking, D.J. and Chilvers, C.E. (1999) 'Habitual physical activity and bone mineral density in postmenopausal women in England', *International Journal of Epidemiology*, vol 28, no 2, pp 241-246.

40 Sarton, M., cited in F.K. Furman (1997) *Facing the mirror: Older women and beauty shop culture*, London: Routledge, p 2.

41 de Beauvoir, S. (1972) *Old age* (trans P. O'Brian), London: Andre Deutsch, p 2.

42 Rowe, DE. (1994) *Time on our side*, London: HarperCollins, pp 36-37.

43 Wilson, G. (1995) '"I'm the eyes and she's the arms": changes in gender roles in advanced old age', in S. Arber and J. Ginn (eds) *Connecting gender and ageing*, Buckingham: Open University Press, p 99.

44 Ginn, J. and Arber, S. (1995) '"Only connect": gender relations and ageing', in Arber and Ginn, p 6.

45 Thompson, P., Itzin, C. and Abendstern, N. (1990) *I don't feel old,* Oxford: Oxford University Press, p 107.

46 Furman, p 3.

47 Alda, A. (1999) *Hurry Granny Annie,* Berkeley, Cal.: Tricycle Press.

48 Cole, B. (2004) *The trouble with Gran,* London: Egmont Books.

49 Hummel, C., Rey, J-C. and D'Epinay, C.J.L. (1995) 'Children's drawings of grandparents', in M. Featherstone and A. Wernick (eds) *Images of ageing: Cultural representations of later life,* London: Routledge.

50 Rowe, p 79.

51 MacDonald, B. with Rich, C. (1984) *Look me in the eye: Old women, ageing and ageism,* London: The Women's Press, p 14.

52 Furman, p 2.

53 de Beauvoir, p 283.

54 Heilbrun, C.G. (1997) *The last gift of time: Life after sixty,* New York: Ballantine Books, p 128.

55 Woolf, V. (1928) *Orlando,* London: The Hogarth Press (1993, Virago), p 199.

56 Hugman, R. (1999) 'Embodying old age', in E.K. Teather (ed.) *Embodied geographies: Space, bodies and rites of passage,* London: Routledge, p 194.

57 Comfort, A. (1977) *A good age,* London: Mitchell Beazley Publishers, p 20.

58 Cited in de Beauvoir, p 298.

59 Lodge, D. (1984) *Small world,* London: Secker and Warburg, p 373.

60 Elias, N. (1985) *The loneliness of the dying* (trans. E. Jephcott), Oxford: Blackwell, p 68.

61 Becker, G. (1997) *Disrupted lives: How people create meaning in a chaotic world,* Berkeley: University of California Press, p 89.

62 Gowing, L. (2003) *Common bodies: Women, touch and power in seventeenth century England,* New York: Yale University Press, p 76.

63 LeGuin, U. (1989) 'The space crone', in *Dancing at the edge of the world,* New York: Harper and Row.

64 Tanne, J.H. (2004) 'Living on cruiseships is cost effective for elderly people', *British Medical Journal,* vol 329, p 1065.

Chapter 8

1   Dreger, A.D. (2004) *One of us: conjoined twins and the future of normal,* Cambridge, Mass.: Harvard University Press, p 40.

2   Murray, C.D. (2001) 'The experience of bodily boundaries by Siamese twins', *New Ideas in Psychiatry,* vol 19, no 2, pp 117-130.

3   Dreger, p 7.

4   Murray, p 119.

5   Bratton, M.Q. and Chetwynd, S.B. (2004) 'One into two will not go: conceptualising conjoined twins', *Journal of Medical Ethics,* vol 30, pp 279-285, p 279.

6   Sacks, O. (1990) *A leg to stand on,* London: HarperCollins, p 202.

7   Bratton and Chetwynd.

8   Murray, p 19.

9   Dreger, p 126.

10 Dreger, p 6.

11 Woodforde, J. (1968) *The strange story of false teeth*, London: Routledge and Kegan Paul.

12 Oakley, A. and Ashton, J. (eds) (1997) *The gift relationship: From human blood to social policy. By Richard M Titmuss*. London: LSE Books.

13 Poole, F.J. (1983) 'Cannibals, tricksters and witches', in P. Brown and D. Trizin (eds) *The ethnography of cannibalism*, Washington, D.C.: Society for Psychological Anthropology.

14 Marrimer, B. (1992) *Cannibalism: The last taboo*, London: Arrow Books.

15 Agrawal, C.M. (1998) 'Reconstructing the human body using biomaterials', *Journal of Materials*, vol 50, no 1, pp 31-5.

16 Shilling, C. (2005) *The body in culture, technology and society*, London: Sage, p 183.

17 Ott, K (2002) 'The sum of its parts', in K. Ott, D. Serlin and S. Milim (eds) *Artifical parts, practical lives*, New York: New York University Press.

18 Milim, S. (2002) '"A limb which shall be presentable in polite society": prosthetic techniques in the nineteenth century', in K. Ott, D. Serlin and S. Milim (eds) *Artifical parts, practical lives*, New York: New York University Press.

19 Serlin, D. (2002) 'Engineering masculinity: veterans and prosthetics after World War Two', in K. Ott, D. Serlin and S. Milim (eds) *Artifical parts, practical lives*, New York: New York University Press.

20 Agrawal.

21 Kimbrell, A. (1993) *The human body shop: The engineering and the marketing of life*, San Francisco: Harper and Row.

22 Goodwin, M. (2006) *Black markets: The supply and demand of body parts,* Cambridge: Cambridge University Press.

23 Becker, A.R. (1994) 'Nurturing and negligence: working on other's bodies', in T.J. Csordas (ed.) *Embodiment and experience,* Cambridge: Cambridge University Press, p 112.

24 Gilman, S.L. (1999) *Making the body beautiful: A cultural history of aesthetic surgery,* Princeton, New Jersey: Princeton University Press, p 309.

25 Blum, V.L. (2003) *Flesh wounds: The culture of cosmetic surgery,* Berkeley, Cal.: University of California Press, p 54.

26 Gilman, pp 6, 35.

27 Blum, p 54.

28 Bordo, S. (2003) *Unbearable weight: Feminism, Western culture and the body,* Berkeley: University of California Press, p xvi.

29 Taylor, S.E. and Langer, E.J. (1977) 'Pregnancy: a social stigma?' *Sex Roles,* vol 3, no 1, pp 27-35.

30 Goffman, E. (1990) *Stigma: Notes on the management of spoiled identity,* London: Penguin.

31 Rothman, B.K. (1988) *The tentative pregnancy,* London: Pandora Press.

32 Longhurst, R. (2001) 'Breaking corporeal boundaries', in R. Holliday and J. Hassard (eds) *Contested bodies,* London: Routledge.

33 Young, M. (1990) *Throwing like a girl and other essays in feminist philosophy and social theory,* Bloomington, Indiana: Indiana University Press, p 163.

34 Davidson, J. (2001) 'Pregnant pauses: agoraphobic embodiment and the limits of (im)pregnability', *Gender, Place and Culture: A Journal of Feminist Geography*, vol 8, no 3, pp 283-297.

35 Faisal-Cury, A. and Menezes, P.R. (2006) 'Factors associated with a preference for Caesarean delivery', *Rev. Saúde Pública*, vol 40, no 2: doi:10.1590/S0034-89102006000200007.

36 Bordo, pp 81-82.

37 Kolder, V.E., Gallagher, J. and Parsons, M.T. (1987) 'Court-ordered obstetrical interventions', *New England Journal of Medicine*, vol 316, no 19, pp 1192-1196.

38 Oakley, A. (1984) *The captured womb*, Oxford: Basil Blackwell.

39 Petechesky, R. (1987) 'Foetal images: the power of visual culture and the politics of reproduction', in M. Stanworth (ed.) *Reproductive technologies: Gender, motherhood and medicine*, Cambridge: Polity Press, p 69.

40 Draper, J. (2002) '"It was a real good show": the ultrasound scan, fathers and the power of visual knowledge', *Sociology of Health and Illness*, vol 24, no 6, pp 771-795.

41 Sandelowksi, M. (1994) 'Separate, but less equal: fetal ultrasonography and the transformation of expectant mother/fatherhood', *Gender and Society*, vol 8, no 2, pp 230-245.

42 Hausman, B. (2004) 'The feminist politics of breastfeeding', *Australian Feminist Studies*, vol 19, no 45, pp 273-285.

43 Hausman.

44 Hausman, p 275.

45 Braidotti, R. (1997) 'Mothers, monsters and machines', in J. Conboy, N. Medina and S. Stanbury (eds) *Writing on the body: Female embodiment and feminist theory*, New York: Columbia University Press, pp 64-65.

Chapter 9

1   Olson, W.K. (1991) *The litigation explosion*, New York: Dutton, p 184.
2   Friedman, L.M. (2002) *American law in the twentieth century,* New Haven: Yale University Press, p 375.
3   Olson, p 5.
4   http://forums.freecovers.net/ index.php?showtopic=515, accessed 28 June 2006.
5   Friedman, p 457.
6   Olson, p 29.
7   Drinker, H.S. (1953) *Legal ethics*, New York: Columbia University Press, p 211.
8   Olson, p 24.
9   Olson, p 9.
10 Olson p 45.
11 Bell, P.A. and O'Connell, J. (1997) *Accidental justice: The dilemmas of tort law,* New Haven: Yale University Press, p 20.
12 Friedman, p 349.
13 Friedman, p 372.
14 Bell and O'Connell, p 16.
15 Buchan, A., Kennedy, J. and Woolf, E. (2003) *Personal injury practice,* London: LexisNexis UK, p 58.
16 Bawden, N. (2005) *Dear Austen,* London: Virago, p 124.
17 Olson, p 112.
18 Bell and O'Connell, p 21.

19 Burdick, L.D. (1905) *The hand: A survey of facts, legends and beliefs pertaining to manual ceremonies, covenants and symbols*, New York: The Irving Company, pp 48-9.

20 Friedman, p 266.

21 Olson, p 9.

22 Bell and O'Connell, p 21.

23 Bell and O'Connell, p 22.

24 Sandbach, J. (2004) *No win, no fee, no chance: CAB evidence in the challenges facing access to injury compensation*, London: CAB, p 13.

25 Gibb, F. (2006) 'Ambulance chasers cast profession in bad light', *The Times*, 7 October.

26 Campos, P.E. (1998) *Jurismania: The madness of American law*, New York: Oxford University Press, p 184, p 182.

Chapter 10

1 Kleinman, A. (1988) *The illness narratives*, New York: Basic Books.

2 Williams, G. (1984) 'The genesis of chronic illness: narrative re-construction', *Sociology of Health and Illness*, vol 6, no 2, pp 175-200.

3 Murphy, R.F. (1987) *The body silent*, London: JM Dent.

4 Dalyell, T. (2006) 'Professor David Simpson: pioneer of powered prosthetic limbs', *The Independent* 23 June.

5 Williams, S.J. and Bendelow, G. (1998) *The lived body: Sociological themes, embodied issues*, London: Routledge.

6 Tan, A.M. (1992) 'Sensibility testing', in B.G. Stanley and S.M. Tribuzi (eds) *Concepts in hand rehabilitation*, Philadelphia: F.A. Davis.

7 Ziguras, C. (2004) *Self care: Embodiment, personal autonomy and the shaping of health consciousness,* London: Routledge.

8 Low, S.M. (1994) 'Embodied metaphors: nerves as lived experience', in T.J. Csordas (ed.) *Embodiment and experience,* Cambridge: Cambridge University Press.

9 Cocteau, J. (1933) *Opium: The diary of an addict,* London: Allen and Unwin (trans. E Boyd), p 50.

INDEX

Index

medical model 72
Medical Research Council scale 78
medical screening 101-4
men
  artificial hormones 100
  medical screening 102
  osteoporosis 103
Mendelssohn, Felix 90
menopause 97-100
mind, and body 32-3, 88-9
mineral body model 104, 105-7
mirrors 110
misoplegia 30
mounds and obstacles ruling 141-2
multiple sclerosis 60-1
Mundurucu Indians 68
Murphy, Robert 68 9, 70, 148

N

nerve-conduction tests 78, 79, 91
nerves 31-44, 77, 152
neurology 90 1
normality 91-2
Nuer 48, 49
numbness 20-1, 76, 84, 93

O

old age 95-6, 106-13
On writing (King) 21
opium addiction 23, 60, 92, 154
organ transplants 118-19
Orlando (Woolf) 111
osteoarthritis 93
osteopenia 104
osteoporosis 97, 100-1, 103-7

P

pain 75-6, 152
palms 81
paralysed hand, The (Brown, quoted in Lamb) 78
patients
  bodies 71
  compliance 8
  illness narratives 60-1, 68-70
  medical screening 101-2
penis 38-9, 44
phantom limbs 43

physiotherapy 20-1, 27, 79, 80-4, 90-1, 92-4
piano 89-90
Piano concerto for the left hand (Ravel) 50
Pillsbury, Gerald 61, 76
pineal gland 73
post menopausal women 97-101
post-traumatic stress disorder 26
pregnancy 121-5, 126
proprioception 42-3, 83-4, 116
prostate cancer 100, 102
protopathic sensation 37-8
Proust, Marcel 95
purse-snatching 17-19

R

Raine, Nancy 19, 22
Ralston, Aron 14-15
rape survival 19, 22-3
Ravel, Maurice 50
re-education 79-80, 92-3
recovery 130, 135
rehabilitation 79-84, 90-1, 92-4
Rehabilitation of hand function (Leont'ev and Zaporozhets) 40-1
retrospective narratization 148
right hand 25-6, 30, 48-51, 52-7, 140
right hand, The (Hertz) 48, 52
Right hand, left hand (McManus) 52-4, 57
right-handedness 47-8
Rivers, W.H.R. 36-40, 82
Rowe, Dorothy 107-8

S

Sacks, Oliver 31-2, 35, 42, 43, 74, 78, 79, 85
Samak, Niran 83-9
San Francisco Chronicle, The 102
Sand, George 99
Sarton, May 70, 107
Scarry, Elaine 75
scars 65-6, 140
Schappell, Lori and Reba 115
Schumann, Robert 50
screening 101-3